Health and Health Care in Modern Britain

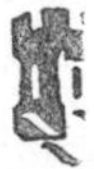

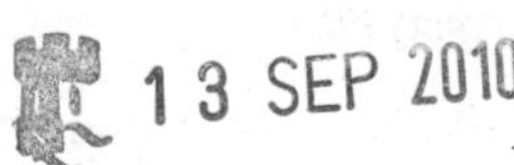

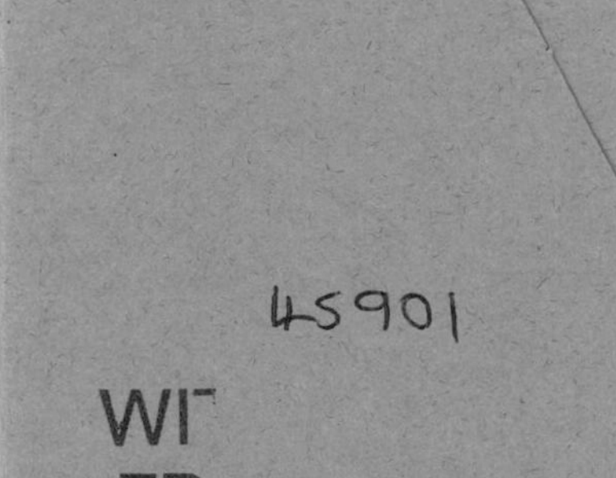

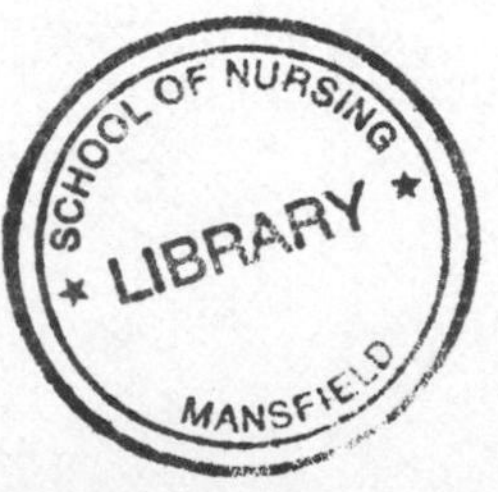

The *Oxford Modern Britain* series comprises authoritative introductory books on all aspects of the social structure of modern Britain. Lively and accessible, the books will be the first point of reference for anyone interested in the state of contemporary Britain. They will be invaluable to those taking courses in the social sciences.

Also published in this series

Kinship and Friendship in Modern Britain
Graham Allen

Religion in Modern Britain
Steve Bruce

Women and Work in Modern Britain
Rosemary Crompton

Mass Media and Power in Modern Britain
John Eldridge, Jenny Kitzinger, and Kevin Williams

Race and Ethnicity in Modern Britain
Second Edition
David Mason

Age and Generation in Modern Britain
Jane Pilcher

Youth and Employment in Modern Britain
Kenneth Roberts

Forthcoming titles

Business and Organization in Modern Britain
Stephen Ackroyd

Nations and Nationalism in Modern Britain
Christopher G. A. Bryant

Gender in Modern Britain
Nickie Charles

Voting Behaviour in Modern Britain
Anthony Heath

Oxford Modern Britain

Health and Health Care in Modern Britain

Joan Busfield

Series Editor: John Scott

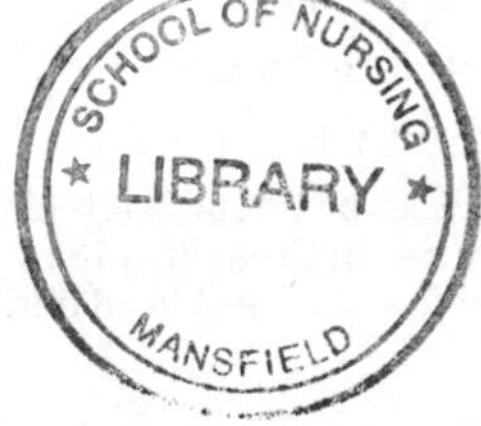

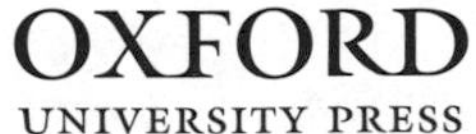

OXFORD
UNIVERSITY PRESS

Great Clarendon Street, Oxford OX2 6DP

Oxford University Press is a department of the University of Oxford.
It furthers the University's objective of excellence in research, scholarship,
and education by publishing worldwide in

Oxford New York

Athens Auckland Bangkok Bogotá Buenos Aires Calcutta
Cape Town Chennai Dar es Salaam Delhi Florence Hong Kong Istanbul
Karachi Kuala Lumpur Madrid Melbourne Mexico City Mumbai
Nairobi Paris São Paulo Singapore Taipei Tokyo Toronto Warsaw

with associated companies in Berlin Ibadan

Oxford is a registered trade mark of Oxford University Press
in the UK and in certain other countries

Published in the United States
by Oxford University Press Inc., New York

British Library Cataloguing in Publication Data
Data available

Library of Congress Cataloging in Publication Data
Data available

ISBN 0-19-878123-7

10 9 8 7 6 5 4 3 2 1

Typeset by RefineCatch Limited, Bungay, Suffolk
Printed in Great Britain by
Biddles Ltd., Guildford and King's Lynn

For my parents

Foreword

THE Oxford Modern Britain series is designed to fill a major gap in the available sociological sources on the contemporary world. Each book will provide a comprehensive and authoritative overview of major issues for students at all levels. They are written by acknowledged experts in their fields, and should be standard sources for many years to come.

Each book focuses on contemporary Britain, but the relevant historical background is always included, and a comparative context is provided. No society can be studied in isolation from other societies and the globalized context of the contemporary world, but a detailed understanding of a particular society can both broaden and deepen sociological understanding. These books will be exemplars of empirical study and theoretical understanding.

Books in the series are intended to present information and ideas in a lively and accessible way. They will meet a real need for source books in a wide range of specialized courses, in 'Modern Britain' and 'Comparative Sociology' courses, and in integrated introductory courses. They have been written with the newcomer and general reader in mind, and they meet the genuine need in the informed public for accurate and up-to-date discussion and sources.

John Scott
Series Editor

Acknowledgements

A NUMBER of colleagues have commented on ealier drafts of various sections of this book. I would like to thank in particular Christopher Bridge of the North East Essex Mental Health NHS Trust, and Charlie Davidson, Sheldon Leader, John Scott (the series editor), and Nigel South of the University of Essex for their helpful comments and advice. I aired some of the ideas in Chapter 6 in papers given in London and Warwick and benefited from the comments of those attending. For academic support and friendship I would like to thank Delfina Dolza, Diana Gittins, and Lydia Morris. Michael Lane, my daughter, Lindsay, and Jeffrey have provided diversion, pleasure, and liveliness as well as support, for which I am much indebted. This book is dedicated to my parents, both now in their late eighties, who provide clear evidence of the gains that can be secured from increases in longevity.

Contents

Contents

Detailed Contents

List of Figures and Tables

Figures

Tables

Chapter 1

The Health of the Nation

THE health of a nation's population, both physical and mental, serves as an excellent barometer of the society's psychological and social well-being. A population that lives long and is relatively free-from ill-health during their lives suggests a society at ease with itself, or, to put the stronger case, a population where illness and incapacity are common and where many people die prematurely, indicates that we can expect to find significant political, social and economic problems within the society as well as personal suffering.

Of course disease and illness are 'natural' processes in a range of senses, not least in that they involve bodily processes. But they are also profoundly social phenomena. On the one hand, these bodily processes are not simply a product of genetic endowment but also of the human organism's relation to the environment—a relation that is shaped by social processes and social organisation. It is for this reason that disease and ill-health, viewed at the level of population, society or nation, are such significant indices of social well-being. Longevity as a summary measure of lifetime biological health is arguably a better and more sensitive indicator of the overall quality of life in a society than economic growth measured in terms of its per capita Gross Domestic Product (Wilkinson 1996: introduction).

On the other hand, health is a social phenomenon, in that the boundaries of health and illness are socially determined and vary across time and place. To say this is not to deny that there is some underlying biological reality to which terms like 'illness' and 'disease' refer. Indeed, the term 'disease' is often taken to refer specifically to objective biological changes; the term 'illness' to the experience of disease (Kleinman 1988: 3–6). It is rather to say that the concepts of disease and illness, which I shall use more or less interchangeably, are often ill-defined and imprecise, and that what is recognized as disease or illness depends on cultural ideas and beliefs and on social institutions (Johansson 1991). Not only do the terms refer variously to suffering, physical lesion, biological malfunctioning, imperfection, statistical abnormality, what doctors treat, and so forth, none of which can be very exactly defined (Kendell 1975), but it is also clear that the precise boundaries of disease and sickness vary across time and place. For instance, in developing countries with high levels of mortality, where most individuals, even young children, must engage in some form of work, where there is no system of state welfare and health services are limited, then symptoms like endemic diarrhoea are not treated as signs of illness (Mull and Mull 1988). Only near-fatal conditions tend to be viewed as illnesses. In more affluent societies, where life expectancy is far higher, the boundaries of illness are usually set more widely and illness thresholds are reduced. In these societies, doctors spend considerable time and money on detecting and identifying new diseases or the earlier stages and signs of illness, and so change the boundaries and thresholds of illness. Put another way, the society subjects disease and illness to a stronger and stronger microscope and in so doing changes what falls within their boundaries. As a result, sickness has a far broader meaning and the tight correlation between levels of mortality and of morbidity—that is, sickness—disappears. This generates a paradox, which I discuss below, that over time as mortality declines—surely a mark of improvements in health—sickness levels appear to *increase*, since economic development is associated with the setting of higher standards of health and lower thresholds of illness.

One consequence is that morbidity data need to be treated with extreme caution. The assumption tends to be that, operating with a definition of health as simply the absence of disease, morbidity data provide some measure of underlying biological health. However, whilst such data *refer* to biological processes, they depend on the thresholds of illness set either by doctors or by the lay population. Another consequence is that the objective of achieving good health for a population in terms both of greater longevity and low levels of sickness may be something of a chimera, since as longevity increases the capacity for identifying and treating problems is also likely to be heightened.

Just as the boundaries and thresholds of illness change over time and place, so the value attached to health varies, since economic and social constraints may make it difficult for a society or social group to attach much importance to health. In that respect good health is a 'luxury' which certain societies and social groups are unable to afford. In an advanced industrial country like Britain, good health comes very high on most people's list of personal desires and there is quite a high degree of health consciousness (Health Education Authority 1996: table 2.20). Indeed, that health is positively valued is integral to the notion itself. To say that a state or condition is one of health is to say it is good or desirable; conversely, to say that a state or condition is one of illness is to say that it is bad or undesirable (King 1954; Sedgwick 1982). In that respect health and illness are essentially evaluative concepts—the former a positive state, the latter a negative one. But this does not mean that good health is equally high on individuals' or a society's agenda. Arguably it often stands higher on the agenda of individuals than on that of governments, who respond intermittently and variably to individuals' priorities. There are also groups and societies (certain groups in the US would be an example) where health consciousness is perhaps excessive, not least because in cultures where health is also seen as an individual responsibility it can lead to blaming and condemning those who become sick.

Though good health is very highly valued by most people in Britain as in other Western societies, precisely what individuals mean by good 'health' varies.[1] The Health and Lifestyles Survey carried out in the mid-1980s identified a range of lay conceptions, including good health as the absence of illness; as energy and vitality; as physical fitness; as having a healthy lifestyle; as psychological fitness; and as the ability to carry out one's normal routines (sometimes termed 'functional health'). When asked about their own health an overwhelming majority defined health in terms either of physical fitness and energy, or of functional health, or of psychological fitness. The survey also showed that conceptions of good health changed with age, and that older age groups, especially men, were more likely to think of health in terms of abilities and functions and less in terms of physical fitness and energy. Overall women were more likely than men to focus on psychological fitness (Blaxter 1990: ch. 2).

Studies also consistently show that spending on health care, which primarily takes the form of services dealing with those who are already sick, is supported by the majority of the population. In Britain, spending on the National Health Service has increased from under 4 per cent of GDP in 1949 to around 6 per cent in 1995–6, but this hides a greater absolute increase in spending over time, since the economy has also expanded considerably over the same period. Yet the NHS regularly tops the list of areas where the public would like to see more public expenditure (ONS 1998b: table 6.21).

Statistics on health care spending need to be deployed with caution. The boundaries of what constitutes health care—that is, activities and interventions explicitly directed towards maintaining health and dealing with sickness—like those of health itself, are not fixed, and in Britain we have been witnessing a period in which the boundary between health and social care has been realigned, primarily at the behest of government, with health care being defined more narrowly in terms of direct, medical involvement, and social care of those with chronic health problems being expanded. Looking after an individual who may be sick or incapacitated but where little active medical intervention is required, or only intermittently, is increasingly being seen as outside the framework of health care. This is because there are financial gains to be secured for the state from redefining the long-term care of chronic sickness as a social not a health matter, since social care, unlike health care, is means-tested.[2]

There is, too, a further caveat about the importance attached to health: that whilst individuals place a high value on health in present-day British society, this does not mean that they necessarily act in ways that maximize their own health, not least because immediate pleasures—for instance drinking and smoking, both known to be linked to long-term health—may take priority over the longer-term goal of the maintenance of health. In practice people quite often act in ways that undermine their health, putting aside the longer-term adverse consequences of some activity, either for the sake of immediate pleasures (including the excitement of risk-taking) or to relieve stress. When so doing they often marshal various psychological strategies to deal with the contradiction between behaviour and attitudes: denying, minimizing, or ignoring the risks, noting counter-instances of the pertinent statistical generalization (long-term smokers who have not developed lung cancer), or asserting the inadequacy of scientific studies (they all show something different). Nor does it mean that the government puts the health of the population especially high on its political agenda. Though the proportion of GDP spent on all types of health care has been increasing, Britain's spending is lower as a proportion of GDP than in several other European countries or in the United States (in 1990 it ranked seventeenth out of twenty-two developed countries: Allsop 1995: 70), and governments often give little attention to the health implications of many other public policies.[3]

What, however, can we establish about the current health of the British population? Are we a relatively healthy nation? Is there much scope for improvement in the population's health? The purpose of this chapter is to consider such questions in some detail. In the following chapter I examine the different types of explanatory account of health and illness, and in Chapter 3 I consider how these accounts can be used to explain the specific differences in health outlined in this chapter.

Long-term trends

Mortality

The long-term trend of sharp reductions in mortality is well known. Viewed in terms of longevity, Britain now has a relatively healthy population in comparison with those of previous centuries. An individual at birth has a much better chance of surviving into old age than a century ago, and if the comparison is with 200 or 300 years ago the differences are even greater. Table 1.1 gives the figures for life expectancy at birth over the period since 1838 (vital registration of births, marriages, and deaths was made statutory in 1837).[4]

The data show the marked increase in life expectancy of both men and women over the last century and a half.[5] For the years 1838–40, men's life expectancy was 40.4 years and women's 42.0; in 1994–6 the comparable figures give a male life expectancy of 74.4 and a female of 79.6 years. The sharp increase in chances of survival is even clearer if we look at the proportions surviving to different ages using the same type of life table data from which life expectancy is calculated. On the basis of 1841 mortality rates, only some 68 per cent of men and 71 per cent of women would survive to the age of 15 (Charlton 1997: 18). Based on 1994–6 mortality data, over 99 per cent of men and women will survive to their 15th birthday. Indeed, 81 per cent of men and 88 per cent of women survive to the age of 65 (far more than survived to 15 150 years ago), and 56 per cent of men and 71 per cent of women to 75 (ONS 1997a: table 2.20).

Table 1.2 gives the figures for infant mortality in England and Wales, another excellent index of a population's health because of its sensitivity to social conditions. It shows how the decline in infant mortality occurred relatively late: it was not until after 1900 that there was a clear trend of reductions in infant mortality, whereas increases in life expectancy were already visible in the nineteenth century; deaths of infants and children are the hardest to reduce.

These dramatic increases in life expectancy and declines in infant mortality are primarily the result of reductions in mortality from infectious diseases,

Table 1.1 Life expectancy of men and women at birth, England and Wales, 1838–1994

	Male	Female		Male	Female
1838–44	40.4	42.0	1930–2	58.7	62.9
1838–54	39.9	41.9	1950–2	68.4	71.5
1871–80	41.4	44.6	1960–2	68.1	74.0
1881–90	43.7	47.2	1970–2	69.0	75.2
1891–1900	44.1	47.8	1981–3*	71.3	77.2
1901–10	48.5	52.4	1990–2	73.4	79.0
1910–12	51.5	55.4	1994–6	74.4	79.6
1920–2	55.6	59.6			

Source: Office of Population Censuses and Surveys, *OPCS Monitor*, DH1 No. 2 table 21 (data from 1838 to 1962 are from the English Life Table; for 1970–2 from the abridged Life Tables); CSO/ONS, *Annual Abstract of Statistics*, 1985; 1995; 1998: table 2.22.

* The Annual Abstract did not provide figures for 1980–2.

Table 1.2 Infant mortality, England and Wales, 1841–1996*

Year	Rate	Year	Rate
1841–50	153	1930–2	64
1851–60	154	1940–2	55
1861–70	154	1950–2	29
1871–80	149	1960–2	22
1881–90	142	1970–2	18
1891–1900	153	1980–2	11
1900–02	146	1990–2	7
1910–12	110	1996	6
1920–22	80		

Source: Office of Population Censuses and Surveys (1978: No. 2. table 4); ONS (1998a: Table 2.20).

* The 19th-c. figures are 10-year averages; figures for this century are 3-year averages except for 1996.

which have tended to exact their highest toll amongst infants and children, who are usually less resistant to infections (those who survived to later ages had increased resistance, though infections killed some adults as well as infants and children). In the nineteenth century the major killers were infectious diseases such as cholera and tuberculosis (TB) and, to a lesser extent, diphtheria, small-pox, measles, and pneumonia. By the middle of this century death rates from these killers were considerably reduced (McKeown 1976), with declines in their incidence and also in the case-fatality rate (the chances that a person who became ill would die).[6] Figure 1.1 shows, for example, the rapid decline in the death rate from TB in Britain between 1860 and 1950.

With the decline in infectious diseases as causes of death, diseases that kill people when they are older have come to prominence. In late modern Britain, as in other advanced industrial societies, the so-called 'degenerative' or non-infectious diseases, which are considered indicative of the body's wearing out (often prematurely), are the major causes of death. The most common are heart diseases, respiratory diseases, and cancers. These are sometimes described as the diseases of affluence since they are the main causes of death in more wealthy societies, but this is an unfortunate appellation since, as we shall see, premature death from these causes is actually more common amongst the poorer sections of society: they are positively associated with economic development but negatively associated with income at a single point of time.

The long-term decline in mortality associated with major changes in the types of disease that cause death is now usually termed the epidemiological

Figure 1.1 Deaths from tuberculosis, Britain, 1860–1950

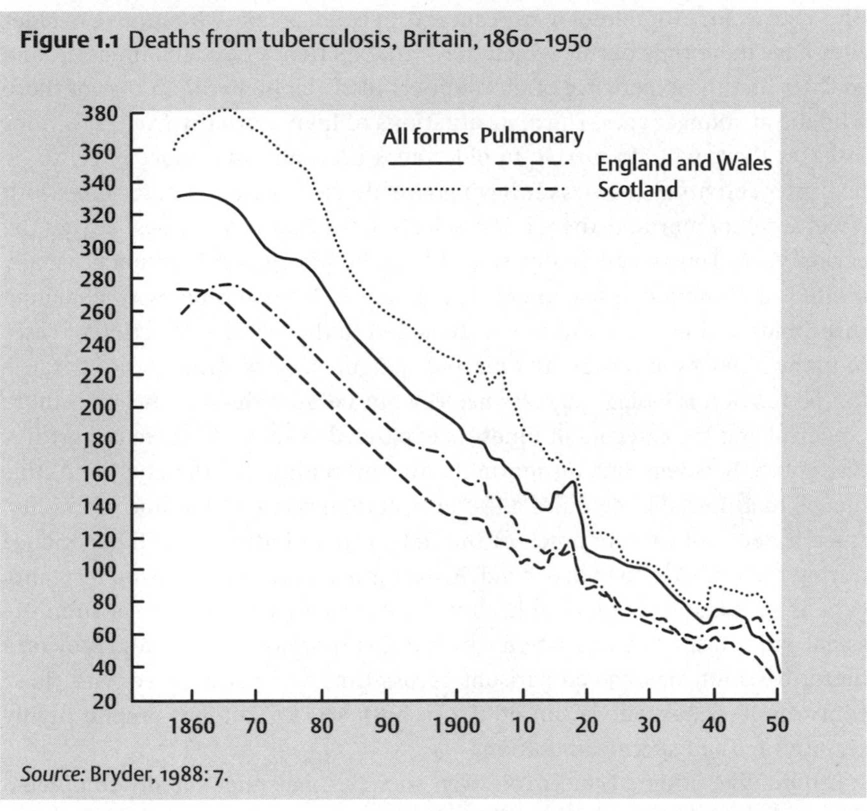

Source: Bryder, 1988: 7.

transition (Omran 1971)—epidemiology being the study of the distribution of diseases.[7] The transition has three key features: (a) a decline in mortality concentrated on infectious diseases, which tend to be displaced by non-infectious diseases; (b) a shift in the burden of illness from younger to older age groups; and (c) a change from a situation dominated by acute, often fatal, illnesses to one in which many people experience illnesses that do not result in death but may become chronic (Frenk et al. 1991). This latter shift from ill-health dominated by mortality to ill-health that is less likely to kill is now commonly termed the 'health transition'; it suggests the paradox to which I have already alluded: in societies where people typically live longer, and in that respect could be said to be healthier, more morbidity is identified.

However, a number of different processes need to be distinguished. First, there is the fact that infectious illnesses when they kill people often do so quickly, although the case-fatality of an infectious disease depends on a range of factors, including the health of the population amongst which it spreads, the methods of treatment available, if any, and so forth. In contrast, non-infectious diseases often lead to a longer period of sickness and incapacity before death (this is true, for example, of many cancers). Second, people who survive to older ages have more time during which they can experience non-fatal illnesses, and so their lifetime experience of morbidity is likely be higher than that of those who die at younger ages. Third, in situations of high mortality from infectious diseases those who do survive to older ages are somewhat more likely to be healthier and fitter (the weaker having already died), whereas in societies with lower levels of mortality there is less selection for health and fitness during the earlier years. Fourth and finally, since the epidemiological transition is usually related to economic development, it is likely to be associated with changing thresholds of illness. New illnesses are added to the list, the detection of cases of many illnesses improves, and morbidity figures are pushed up, not because the population is biologically less healthy but because the microscope is more powerful and the category of illness is expanded. As a result there is a greater divergence between data on mortality and morbidity. On the one hand, this means that mortality becomes a less adequate measure of lifetime morbidity, since it does not capture much of the ill-health an individual will experience during their life. On the other hand, it strengthens the case for using mortality data as a measure of biological health, since the data are rather freer from the social and cultural contamination which inflict morbidity data and so provide a better basis for making comparisons across time and place. Faced with these contrary pressures, all we can do is use both sets of data but remain highly sensitive to their specific limitations.

Britain, like other advanced Western societies, has undoubtedly completed the epidemiological transition. Though data on the causes of death are not especially reliable (Prior 1985), it is clear that the main causes of death in Britain are now, as I have already noted, heart disease, cancers, and respiratory diseases (infectious agents are implicated in some of these diseases). Changes in the age profile of mortality during this century show the greatest reductions in mortality occurring at the earliest ages. The age-specific death rates for the period 1931 to 1987 are given in Table 1.3.

The data show clearly the decline in mortality at all ages, with proportionate declines particularly high in childhood; they also show the way in which, apart from the first year of life, mortality is now very low until one moves into the 45–54 age group. Significantly, too, life expectancy is continuing to increase even for those aged 65 and over. Whereas mortality data for 1972–6 yielded a life expectancy of 12.3 years for men at 65 and for women of 16.2 years, on the basis of 1987–91 data male life expectancy at 65 was 13.5 years and female 17.2 (Hattersley 1997: tables 6.1 and 6.5).

Table 1.3 Age-specific death rates by gender, England and Wales, 1931–1987

	0	1–4	5–14	15–24	25–34	35–44	45–54	55–64	65–74	75+
Males										
1931	79.8	8.1	1.9	2.9	3.4	5.7	11.5	23.9	58.8	155.2
1951	34.0	1.5	0.6	1.1	1.6	2.9	8.6	24.1	59.1	154.6
1971	19.8	0.8	0.4	0.9	1.0	2.3	5.3	13.1	37.0	127.2
1987	10.7	0.4	0.2	0.8	0.9	1.7	5.0	16.0	41.2	110.2
Females										
1931	59.3	7.0	1.7	2.6	3.3	4.5	8.3	17.7	44.3	134.5
1951	25.8	1.3	0.4	0.8	1.3	2.3	5.3	13.1	37.0	127.2
1971	15.1	0.6	0.3	0.4	0.6	1.6	4.3	20.2	26.5	100.3
1987	8.1	0.4	0.2	0.3	0.5	1.1	3.2	9.1	22.8	83.0

Rates per 1,000 population

Source: Illsley et al. (1991: table A4)

Morbidity

Measured in terms of mortality there can be no doubt, therefore, that the population in Britain is far healthier than it was at the beginning of the century. What, however, of the situation in terms of morbidity? Not surprisingly, given what I have said about the fluidity of the category of illness and the way standards of health change over time, we do not have reliable aggregate data on morbidity over the long-term that are independent of measures of mortality. We can, however, look at recent data on morbidity and compare it with the picture we gain from data on mortality. Morbidity can be measured in a number of different ways. A key distinction is between assessments made by clinicians, arguably a more objective measure of sickness and disease, and those based on individual self-reports either of their own state of health or of the presence or absence of various symptoms or incapacities. The term 'incapacity' here is used to refer to the lack of ability, usually as a result of illness or some bodily impairment, to perform an activity in the range considered normal, and is chosen over the stronger term 'disability', which also suggests a permanency to the incapacity.[8]

The General Household Survey collects data on self-reported illness as well as on visits to doctors. In 1996, over one-third of men (34 per cent) and women (35 per cent) reported they had some form of long-standing (i.e. chronic) illness, the percentages increasing markedly with age, from 27 per cent amongst those aged 16–44 to 66 per cent of those aged 75 and over. In response to a further question as to whether their long-standing illness limited their activities (i.e. more a measure of incapacities) some 23 per cent of women and 21 per cent of men reported 'limiting' long-standing illness. The data are given in Table 1.4, which also includes the percentages reporting that they restricted activities in the last 14 days due to illness (more a measure of acute than chronic illness).

The data show the same association with age as the mortality data: age, as we might expect, being positively associated with higher morbidity in the form of chronic, though not acute, illness (except amongst those aged 75 and over). It is possible that this positive association could be partly due to older people, who tend to give health a somewhat higher priority, setting lower thresholds for chronic illness and incapacity (as I noted earlier, they tend to think of health in more functional terms). However, there is evidence that older people often describe themselves as healthy despite having symptoms of chronic illness and incapacity (Blaxter 1990: 32), and little evidence that setting lower thresholds is a significant factor. It seems reasonable to conclude that, as we normally assume, as people age there are increasing signs that their bodies are wearing out, and that typically they face more chronic illnesses and incapacities, many of which are not fatal but some of which may eventually prove to be. The contrast with the long-term trends is striking. For a range of reasons, over the long term reductions in mortality tend, as I have noted, to be *inversely* associated with higher observed levels of morbidity, both acute and chronic, with a key role being played by the emergence of lower

Table 1.4 Long-standing illness, limiting long-standing illness, and restricted activity by age, Britain, 1996

	Long-standing illness		Limiting long-standing illness		Restricted activity	
	M	F	M	F	M	F
0–4	14	13	4	4	12	9
5–15	19	16	8	8	10	9
16–44	27	27	14	16	13	15
45–64	46	47	31	32	18	22
65–74	61	58	42	40	19	21
75 and over	64	68	50	53	23	25
Total	34	35	21	23	15	15

Source: (ONS 1998b: table 8.1)

thresholds of illness associated with deploying a stronger and stronger medical microscope.

Further evidence for changing illness thresholds over time is provided by trends in the General Household Survey (GHS) data since its inception which show increases in all three measures of illness. In 1972, when the first GHS health data were collected, only 21 per cent reported long-standing illness compared with 35 per cent in 1996, and 8 per cent reported restricted activity compared with 16 per cent in 1996. In 1975, the first year when data were collected on 'limiting' long-standing illness, 15 per cent reported this, whereas the 1996 figure was 22 per cent (ONS 1998b: table 8.1). Part of this increase in self-reported illness is due to the changing age structure of the population (as more people fall into the higher age bands the aggregate figure for the whole population is pushed up), but this is not sufficient to account for all the rise, and in the case of limiting illness the increases have occurred particularly amongst the under-65s. Consequently, the data are consistent with, and provide some support for, the view that over time thresholds of illness are lowered (during the same period life expectancy increased by around three years)—a view further supported by the fact that there have been increases over time in the levels of acute as well as chronic sickness.

The positive association between age and chronic illness and incapacity suggests a picture of increases in longevity that enable most people to survive into old age, but of increases bought at the price not only of more instances of acute illness throughout one's lifetime, surely an acceptable price for most people, but also for many of long periods of chronic illness and incapacity during old age. This, of course, raises the question of whether the gains in longevity over recent years are simply additional years of illness. Using GHS data it is possible to calculate a healthy life span for men and women, as well as the number of years of sickness (measured in terms of limiting long-standing illness). Using 1994 data, men's healthy life expectancy was 59.7 years out of a total life expectancy of 74.3 years, and women's 62.2 out of 79.6 years. This suggests that of women's extra five and a half years of life, on average three are spent with chronic sickness. From this it might be inferred that the gains from greater longevity are rather small, a conclusion also suggested by analysis of changes in life expectancy and healthy life expectancy over the period since 1976. In this period men's life expectancy has increased 4.3 years and their healthy life expectancy only 1.8; women's life expectancy has increased 3.5 years and their healthy life expectancy by only 0.2 (ONS 1998c: table 7.5). However, this is an extremely complex and contested area (see Caselli and Lopez 1996). It is important to recognize that the data on healthy life expectancy are constructed from the responses to questions on limiting long-standing illness in the GHS, and I have already noted that the increase in this category of illness is almost certainly affected by changing illness thresholds.

A major issue is trying to disentangle the effect of age from 'proximity to death': is there typically a period of chronic sickness and disability prior to death in old age whether it occurs at, say, 70 or at 80?[9] Or is it that, as longevity increases, there is little or no increase in healthy life expectancy? Certainly one needs not only to distinguish between acute and chronic illness, but also between the levels of severity of the illness or incapacity. Some of the limiting long-standing illnesses that people report in the GHS include conditions like asthma, angina, and high blood pressure, whose symptoms can be kept under control quite well. And some, as I have already argued, arises from better detection and lower illness thresholds. It properly falls into the category of illness as now constituted, but in earlier decades it might not. Clearly, we want the later years of life to be as free as possible from the burden of sickness, pain, and incapacity. But we should not overstate the case about the burden of sickness experienced in old age and assume that there is or can be no gain for most people from greater longevity. Of course, the quality of an older person's life is not just a matter of their health but also of their living environment, resources, and social networks (all of which also affect their health), and in a society where those who reach retirement age often feel they have too little to contribute and are more likely to experience poverty (Arber and Ginn 1991), the gains from greater longevity may be double-edged.

The rather optimistic picture of improving health generated by focusing on mortality data has therefore to be modified once we look at the data on morbidity, which suggest a more complex picture of increases in reported sickness with age, though not one untypical of advanced industrial societies. This might therefore suggest there are still some grounds for satisfaction about long-term improvements in the health of the British population. This may well be so. Nonetheless, a range of other data suggests that there is little cause for complacency. Indeed, there are features of the health of the population almost invisible in the aggregate picture I have described so far that amount to no less than a social scandal because of the pain, misery, and suffering resulting from ill-health and premature mortality, both for those who are sick and for their families and friends, a scandal that only the wilful blindness of the powerful has allowed to continue.

What aspect of health and illness in Britain should generate greater concern and action? Why should we be far from satisfied with the nation's health?

International comparisons

First, we can compare Britain's health record with that of other countries. Here we find that Britain is by no means top of the league in terms of the standard indicators: life expectancy and infant mortality. Of the twenty-five European countries listed in the World Health Organization's *World Health Report 1995* which met their three health targets (including an average life expectancy of at least 60), nine, including Greece, Italy, Spain, France, and Switzerland, had a higher life expectancy in 1993 than the UK's 76—a figure (the figures are rounded) equal to that of five other European countries. Britain's figure was the same as that of the US, but below that of Canada, Australia, and Japan, which in 1993 had the highest life expectancy of all at 79 years (WHO 1995: table A1). The study reported infant mortality in Britain in 1993 at 8 per 1,000 live births.[10] This is quite a low figure (the same as for the US) but still higher than that of countries such as Canada, Denmark, Germany, France, Iceland, Singapore, and Japan—the country with the lowest figure, with only 5 deaths per 1,000 live births (again, nine European countries had lower rates than Britain).

Another set of comparative data was presented in the Green Paper *Our Healthier Nation* (Secretary of State for Health, 1998a). This compared life expectancy in England with that in fourteen other European Union countries around 1995 (Secretary of State for Health, 1998a: fig. 6). Male life expectancy in England ranked sixth at 74.3 years (0.3 years higher than the EU average); female life expectancy, though higher than men's, ranked tenth at 79.5 years, compared with an EU average of 80.7 years (Sweden, followed by Greece, the Netherlands, Italy, and France, had the highest male, and France, Sweden, Spain, Italy, and Luxemburg the highest female life expectancy). Moreover, Britain's international position is declining, and it is not making the gains in longevity achieved elsewhere.[11] It also needs to be noted that the life expectancy figures are based on period mortality data, and so in part reflect the social and economic conditions that individuals who die in a particular year may have experienced long before (some in the early decades of the century). We do not know whether those alive in Britain today, especially those who are still very young, will achieve the same life expectancy as those who died in the period 1994–6.

International comparisons of morbidity are far less reliable than data on mortality, but some of the comparisons indicate key areas where Britain's health record is poor. For instance, comparisons show that levels of heart disease are particularly high in Britain, especially in Scotland.[12] Significantly, too, recent European data indicate that survival rates for some cancers, such as breast cancer, are lower in Britain than elsewhere in Europe (this has been attributed to the comparative lack of specialist oncology services in Britain).

New or expanding problems

This leads to the second area where there is cause for concern: the evidence of new or expanding areas of morbidity as well as some signs that the health of the population may actually be deteriorating rather than improving. It is well known that the population overall was healthier and fitter during the Second World War and the immediate postwar period than previously, and notwithstanding the casualties of war the gains in life expectancy during the 1940s were spectacular (see Table 1.1). The reasons for this are debated and are discussed further in Chapters 2 and 3. Yet there tends to be little recognition of the fact that the health of the present-day population may not have been improving over the last two decades, even though life expectancy based on current mortality but reflecting past social conditions is continuing to increase at present. Certainly, some health scares, such as those surrounding AIDS, new variant Creutzfeldt–Jakob disease (CJD) and E-coli dominate the media from time to time, but their significance for the overall health of the population is rarely examined. Yet cumulatively they raise serious questions about the nation's health, and in some cases their effects are more likely to surface in future mortality data (for instance, the average length of time between being infected by the HIV virus and dying from AIDS is currently around ten years; the incubation of CJD is also long).

Which signs of ill-health now give cause for concern? One is the re-emergence of infectious diseases once considered to have been more or less brought under control. Although statistics on specific diseases raise problems of reliability, there is evidence that TB is returning, albeit at present at quite low levels (Galbraith and McCormick 1997: 9).[13] This is significant, since TB, like infant mortality, is regarded as a good index of social and economic conditions. Other infectious diseases such as meningitis have also increased recently (p. 11). Another sign is the new infectious diseases many associated with the media scares that I have already mentioned. These include AIDS, which first came into public consciousness in the 1980s, CJD associated with BSE in cattle, E-coli and salmonella, both also food-related diseases, cases of which have increased markedly over recent years, and Legionnaire's disease, transmitted by droplets of water. In some cases the media have exaggerated the threat to the nation's health, and figures of the likely number of cases have had to be scaled down (AIDS in Western but not Third World societies is the most obvious example of exaggerated predictions), but frequently there is clear evidence of an increase in the particular disease in question (Galbraith and McCormick 1997: 27).

Another sign of possible deterioration in the health of the population is the increase in various forms of allergies. Asthma, which is certainly exacerbated by air pollution though probably not caused by it, has been increasing in recent years (Marks and Burney 1997: 104–5), as have allergies such as hay fever, and the evidence indicates that these increases are not simply the product of improvements in detection but represent a real increase in incidence. Mental health is a further area of concern. Here it is even harder to be certain that any increases in the number of cases of mental illness that come to medical attention reflect a real deterioration in mental health, though some commentators argue strongly that this is so (e.g. James 1997). Part of the problem is that health service developments as well as changes in treatment (most obviously the revolution in psychotropic medications) have made it much more likely that mental health problems will be brought to professional attention, so that thresholds have changed. Moreover, cultural changes are almost certainly affecting the ways in which tensions and stresses in people's lives are expressed, as well as the willingness to admit to psychological problems, so that what might once have been given somatic form in a physical illness is now more likely to be given psychological expression and is reflected in changed self-perceptions of mental well-being. What is clear, however, is that mental health problems brought to professional attention are on the increase, especially depression. This is also true of problems sometimes categorized as mental health and sometimes as deviance such as drug addiction and alcoholism, though it is hard to establish long-term trends.[14] However, the number of addicts known to the Home Office has increased from under 1,500 in 1970 to over 37,000 in 1995 (Plant 1997: 123), and average alcohol consumption has increased significantly in the postwar period (plant 116). One area where the evidence is a little more clear-cut is that of suicide.[15] Suicides of men aged 15–44 rose steadily over the 1970s and 1980s, but have declined a little during the 1990s (those of women aged 15–44 have declined steadily since 1980: Secretary of State for Health 1998a: fig. 11).

In addition to these increases in specific illnesses, a number of changes in risk factors are likely to be portents of illness to come and may well show up in mortality data in twenty or thirty years' time.[16] Notable here is the marked increase in obesity since the beginning of the 1980s. Obesity increases the risk of heart disease through its association with raised blood pressure and plasma cholesterol (Secretary of State for Health 1992: 55), and the *Health of the Nation* report noted that 8 per cent of men and 12 per cent of women aged 16–64 were obese in 1986/7. Since then the National Audit Office's progress report on the Health of the Nation targets showed that obesity had further increased in both men (to 13 per cent) and women (to 16 per cent) (National Audit Office 1996: 20–1).[17] Levels of exercise are also falling quite dramatically because of the changing character of paid work, the development of new technologies in the home, and new forms of transport, and this is likely to have long-term health consequences. Another worrying sign is that, whilst the long-term trends in smoking across the population have been favourable, it is increasing amongst the key 11–15 age group (National Audit Office, 1996: 33–4). Drinking is also increasing, particularly amongst women (p. 25), and illicit drug use, which can have adverse effects on health, has also been increasing amongst young people. In 1996 nearly a half of young people aged 16–24 had tried some illicit drug (ONS 1998c: table 7.19). In addition, a substantial decline in the male sperm count over past decades has been noted in Britain and other European countries, and problems of infertility are increasing for this and other reasons.

There are, of course, some signs of improvements in health in the population in recent years. Male mortality rates from lung cancer have been declining steadily over the last three decades and, after increasing in the 1950s and 1960s, female rates have stabilised (Secretary of State for Health 1998a: fig. 12). The National Audit Office's 1996 progress report showed improvements in relation to the targets for coronary heart disease and strokes, lung cancer for men under 75 (but not women), and accidents (1996: table 3). Nonetheless, viewed overall the signs of possible deterioration in the population's health are worrying.

Yet the biggest scandal concerning the nation's health is revealed through an examination of the distribution of health and illness across the population. Ill-health is not randomly distributed but manifests a very marked social patterning. There are major inequalities in health in relation to social class, gender, and ethnicity—inequalities which, as we shall see in Chapter 3, are squarely a matter of social and economic conditions and social relations, and which reveal the full extent of avoidable ill-health and suffering. The best-known and most controversial of these are the social-class inequalities in health.

Inequalities in health

Social class

Whatever the precise formulation of the concept of social class and however it is measured, class differences in health in Britain are very striking and have increased over the past twenty years.[18] The most influential postwar study of class inequalities, the *Black Report*, was commissioned by the Labour Government in 1976 and first published in 1979 (Townsend and Davidson 1988). Using 1971 mortality data and the Registrar-General's measure of social class, it showed that mortality levels for both men and women of working age in the lowest social class were two and a half times higher than those in the highest social class—an enormous difference. The data are given in Table 1.5.

Table 1.5 Death rates and ratios by social class, 15–64 years, England and Wales, 1971

Class	Men	Women	Ratio M/F
I	3.98	2.15	1.85
II	5.54	2.18	1.94
III non-manual	5.80	2.76	1.96
III manual	6.08	3.41	1.78
IV	7.96	4.27	1.87
V	9.88	5.31	1.86
Ratio V/I	2.5	2.5	

Death rates per 1,000 population

Source: Townsend and Davidson (1988: table 1)

According to the 1971 census, the percentage of economically active men falling into the different social classes was: Class I, 5.0 per cent; Class II, 18.2 per cent; Class III, 50.5 per cent; Class IV, 18.0 per cent; and Class V, 8.4 per cent (Townsend and Davidson 1988: appendix, table 1). This means that only 1 in 20 men were experiencing the highest levels of health as measured by mortality data.

There are a number of methodological problems associated with data like these. In the first place, the information on occupation is obtained from death certificates and can be vague and imprecise. Moreover, for men this is the last occupation held, which may well differ from the job they held during most of their lifetime that would often be more crucial to their health. And until recently women's death certificates gave the husband's occupation if they were married and their own only if they were not. Consequently a hybrid system of occupational classification has usually been used to allocate women to social classes. Married women have been classified by their husband's occupations, and the rest according to their own. Subsequent analyses of other data indicate that if all women had been classified according to their own occupations (the class distribution of women's occupations is rather different from men's) the class differences in mortality for women would have been a little smaller (Arber 1989). Arber advocates allocating individuals to social classes on the basis of the occupationally 'dominant' member of the household, man or woman, a method, however, which produces similar class differences in health to that used in the *Black Report*.

That class inequalities in health are not simply a product of the ways in which class is measured is demonstrated by recent analyses using a new socio-economic classification (SEC) produced for the Office for National Statistics. Like the Registrar-General's schema, which has been criticized as having no clear conceptual foundations, it is based on occupation, but in this case groups occupations according to employment relations and conditions (Rose and O'Reilly 1998). The new schema allocates individuals to seven or eight classes (Class 8 covers the never worked or unemployed) instead of five, and yields a far more even distribution of individuals across classes (19 per cent fall into class 1 and 15 per cent into class 2 (Rose and O'Reilly 1998: 35). It has been used in a recent analysis of mortality data from the ONS Longitudinal Survey (Bartley et al. 1998), in which hazard ratios for mortality were calculated for the eight social classes. The figures are given in Table 1.6. Notwithstanding the more even distribution of individuals across classes, the analysis broadly confirms the picture set out in the *Black Report*, though the use of hazard ratios rather than standardized mortality ratios helps to reduce the size of the class differences.

Whilst many of the class analyses concentrate on deaths amongst those of working age, other data show that class inequalities extend throughout the life cycle, not just the 15–64 age range. For example, even amongst those who reach 75 there are still significant class differences in mortality, with men of 75 and over in the lowest social class having a 50 per cent higher death rate than those in the highest social class (Fox and Benzeval 1995).

As we might expect given these class differences in mortality, there are also sharp differences in levels of sickness and disability between social classes, which match the mortality data in being negatively associated with social class.

Table 1.6 Hazard ratios for mortality for 1986–1995 by SEC, men aged 15–64

SEC	Hazard ratio *
1. Higher managerial and professional	0.69
2. Lower managerial and professional	0.94
3. Intermediate employees	0.91
4. Self-employed	0.90
5. Lower supervisors, craft and related	1.04
6. Employees in semi-routine occupations	1.12
7. Employees in routine occupations	1.30
8. Never worked/long-term unemployed	1.38

Source: Bartley et al. (1998)

* Adjusted for age in 5-year bands

They provide further confirmation of the class differences in health, since in this case the figures are not reliant on data on occupation obtained from death certificates. For instance, the *Black Report* identified clear class differences in morbidity. It noted that rates of limiting long-standing illness in the GHS were three times as high amongst male unskilled manual workers as amongst professional men; in women the difference was even greater at 3.2 times as high in the highest compared with the lowest social group. The data are given in Table 1.7.

Since we might expect the more affluent to have, if anything, higher standards of health and lower thresholds of illness, the data on morbidity support the claim that there are marked inequalities in health by social class, and that the differences in mortality outlined above are not simply the product of measurement artefact. Indeed, a recent study carried out in Norway, which tested the hypothesis that the greater reporting of illness by working class men could be due to their over-reporting of illness, compared the answers to questions about long-standing illness from middle- and working-class men who reported such illnesses. It found that working-class men's answers were more realistic—they reported their illnesses as more serious and the evidence indicated that this was the case (Elstad 1996).

Other studies have provided further evidence of class differences in morbidity. The Health and Lifestyles Survey (Blaxter 1990) carried out in 1985–6 provided a range of data showing marked class differences in health. Figure 1.2 shows the sharp class gradient for both men and women for inadequate respiratory function. There are also class gradients for height, blood pressure

Table 1.7 Limiting long-standing illness by socio-economic group, England and Wales, 1971–1972

Socio-economic group	Men	Women
Professional	79	81
Managerial	119	115
Intermediate	143	140
Skilled manual	141	135
Semi-skilled manual	168	203
Unskilled manual	236	257
Ratio unskilled to professional	3.0	3.2

Rates per 1,000 population

Source: General Household Survey in Townsend and Davidson (1988: 55)

Figure 1.2 Class, gender and poor respiratory function*

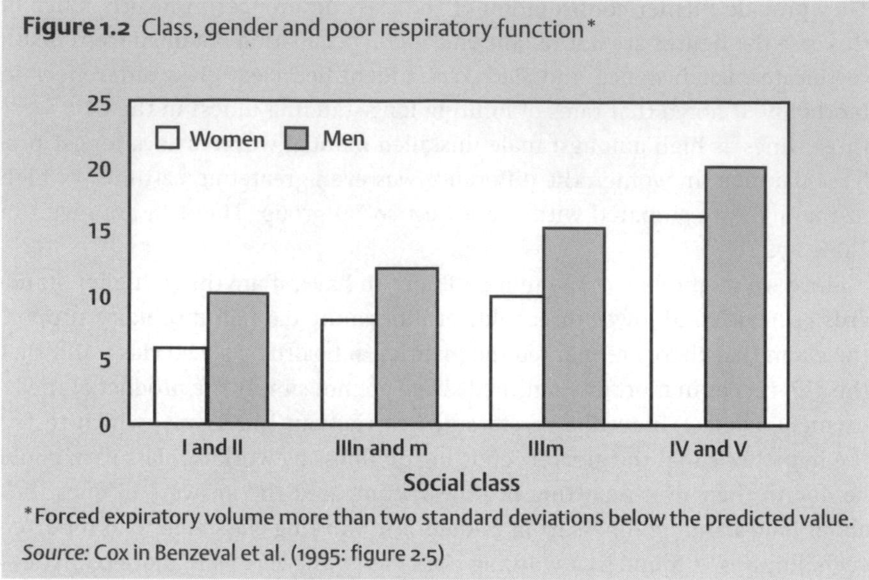

*Forced expiratory volume more than two standard deviations below the predicted value.

Source: Cox in Benzeval et al. (1995: figure 2.5)

and cardiovascular disorder (White et al. 1993) and for mental illness. Rates of psychotic disorder are especially high amongst those in the lowest social class, alcohol and drug dependence in the bottom two social classes, and neurotic disorders in those with lower-status non-manual and manual work (Meltzer et al. 1995: 82). There is also a sharp class gradient in accidents during childhood (Secretary of State for Health 1998a: 65)

The linkage between class and health has been established in a wide range of studies and cannot be simply due to measurement error. Nor does it simply result from processes of social selection in which those with poorer physical and mental health drift down the social scale or have more difficulty in improving their social position. Whilst downward drift does occur, it is not sufficient to account for the widely established links between social class and health. Blane et al. (1993) note, for example, that whilst there is evidence that those with chronic bronchitis may experience some downward mobility during the course of their illness, which tends to be lengthy, this is not possible with lung cancer, since death occurs more quickly; yet the class gradients are essentially the same for the two conditions.

There is also evidence that, after a period following the Second World War when they declined, class inequalities have actually been increasing since the early 1970s (Whitehead 1988; Benzeval et al. 1995; Drever and Whitehead 1997). The difference in life expectancy at birth between men in the two upper and two lower social classes was 2.5 years in the period 1972–6; it was 5.2 years in 1987–91. The data are given in Table 1.8. During the twenty-year period average male life expectancy increased by 3.1 years, but the gains for upper two classes at 3.2 years were far greater than for the lower two social classes at only 0.5 years, despite the latter's lower starting base, which other things being equal would suggest more scope for improvements in life expectancy (the gains for Class III non-manual were highest of all).

The picture for women shows rather smaller class differences, but like those for men they have increased over time, as Table 1.9 shows. Women's average gains in longevity over the twenty-year period at 2.8 years have been smaller than men's, in this case a finding in line with the fact that the base was already higher. However, as with men, the gains for the upper two classes at 3.1 years are greater than for the bottom two at 2.1 years (though the class difference in gain is smaller than for men).

Table 1.8 Life expectancy of men at birth by social class, 1972–91

Social class	1972–6	1977–81	1982–6	1987–91
I and II	71.7	72.8	74.1	74.9
III non-manual	69.5	70.8	72.2	73.5
III manual	69.8	70.0	71.4	72.4
IV and V	69.2	68.3	69.8	69.7
All	69.2	70.0	71.4	72.3
Difference in years between I, II and IV, V	2.5	3.5	4.3	5.2

Source: Hattersley (1997: table 6.1)

Table 1.9 Life expectancy of women at birth by social class, 1972–91

Social class	1972–6	1977–81	1982–6	1987–91
I and II	77.1	78.2	78.7	80.2
III non-manual	78.0	78.1	78.6	79.4
III manual	75.1	76.1	77.1	77.6
IV and V	74.7	75.7	76.8	76.8
All	75.1	76.3	77.1	77.9
Difference in years between I, II and IV, V	2.4	2.5	2.9	3.4

Source: Hattersley (1997: table 6.5)

Morbidity data over time show a somewhat different picture. GHS data indicate that as the levels of reported limiting long-standing illness have increased over time, class differences have become smaller, with the gap declining more for women than men (Bunting 1997: 201). However, in relation to both mortality or morbidity it needs to be remembered that there have been changes in the class structure over the postwar period as a result of changes in the economy.[19] There is evidence, for instance, that the proportions in Class I and II (as measured by the Registrar-General's classification) increased between the 1981 and 1991 censuses and that of all other classes correspondingly declined, but these changes cannot account for the size of the changes in the longevity data presented here.[20]

Others have pointed out that occupational measures of class differences in mortality and morbidity underestimate socio-economic differences in health between social groups since they are based on rather heterogeneous social groups (Wilkinson 1986a). More differentiated measures of social position which compare greater extremes of wealth and poverty yield larger differences. One review concluded that overall there is a difference in life expectancy between the most and least privileged groups of eight years (Fox and Benzeval 1995: 17). A study by Phillimore et al. (1994) of people living in the poorest and richest 10 per cent of electoral wards in the north of England yielded death rates four times as high in the poorest wards. This study circumvented one of the problems of studies linking class to mortality, since it did not depend on the details of occupation obtained from death certificates. Another study (Graham and Blackburn 1998) showed that the length of time on income support was a much better indicator of disadvantage than social class.

Class differences in mortality and morbidity are not, of course, new. In the nineteenth century the social structure of Britain was very different, with most men working either in agriculture or in the new industries, and far fewer non-manual jobs. But the class differences in mortality were striking. Edwin Chadwick, a Poor Law Commissioner, in his 1842 *Report on the Sanitary Condition of the Labouring Population*, set out the average age of death of different occupational groups in two areas, Rutlandshire and Manchester (see Table 1.10).

The data indicate that mortality was far higher in the country than the city—more or less double; they also show that the class differences were almost as extreme. In Manchester, the average age of death amongst the gentry and professional groups at 38 years was over twice that of labourers at 17 years. In Rutlandshire, where overall life expectancy was higher, the difference was somewhat smaller—52 years compared with 38 years—but nonetheless large. Such data do, however, need to be treated with caution

Table 1.10 Average age at death of families by class

	Average age of death (years)	
	Manchester	Rutlandshire
Professional persons, gentry, and families	38	52
Tradesmen and their families*	20	41
Mechanics, labourers, and their families	17	38

Source: Chadwick (1965 [1842]: 223)

* In Rutlandshire farmers and graziers are included with shopkeepers.

(Wohl 1983: 5). Although they relate to a period when vital registration had been introduced (albeit only five years earlier), they do not take account of age differences in the composition of the population and they may well have exaggerated occupational differences in mortality. Yet there can be little doubt that in the mid-nineteenth century the health of the labouring population was poor, and infant and child mortality amongst their families was very high.

Studies earlier this century also highlighted the marked class inequalities in mortality (Stevenson 1923) and the very poor health of some social groups in Britain. Margery Spring Rice's vivid account of working-class women's lives in the 1930s *Working Class Wives: Their Health and Conditions* (1981 [1939]) documented the very poor health of many working-class women drawing on a range of information, including their self-reports in response to a questionnaire, sometimes filled in with the help of a health visitor, and the researchers' own observations. The survey identified 31 per cent (390) of the sample of 1,250 women as in a grave condition of ill-health, and a further 13 per cent (190) as in bad health on the basis of these reports, and Spring Rice was convinced that the women were not exaggerating their ill-health. The most commonly reported problems were anaemia (in nearly half the sample), headaches, constipation with or without haemorrhoids, rheumatism, gynaecological problems, cavernous teeth and toothache, varicose veins, ulcerated legs, and phlebitis. Other ailments included backache, gastric problems, weak eyes, neuralgia, and asthma. Here is her description of one woman's health:

Mrs L.C. of Cardiff says she has been ailing since marriage. She was a housemaid in private service before and was never ill. She is now 39. She has had six children (all still living at home) and one miscarriage; she has a fair house but no bathroom or hot water which she misses 'sadly'. She is badly constipated and has piles and has had backache 'ever since her first confinement which was a difficult one'. She now has also palpitation and cardiac pains. For none of these has she consulted anyone. (Spring Rice 1981: 79).

Class inequalities in health are not, of course, specific to Britain (see Benzeval et al. 1995: 2–3), but that does not make them more acceptable. Moreover there are two reasons for especial concern about the current class inequalities in Britain. First, they are larger than in some other European countries (Whitehead and Diderichson 1997: 63), though those in the US are even greater; second, the class differences in health have been increasing rather than decreasing, in line with sharp increases in income inequalities over the past twenty years unparalleled amongst the countries examined (Atkinson in Benzeval et al. 1995: 1).[21] The high levels of ill-health and mortality in the lower classes not only reveal high levels of pain, suffering, and misery caused by ill-health and premature death amongst these groups, they also play a part in depressing the overall level of health in Britain. Marked inequalities are not only socially and politically unacceptable, they are also a measure of what could be achieved in improved aggregate measures of health.

Gender

Gender inequalities in life expectancy in Britain are also very marked. The data in Tables 1.8 and 1.9 above show a difference in life expectancy between men and women of 5.6 years based on mortality data for 1987–91, with women living to 77.9 years on average and men only to 72.3. This gender difference is not quite as large as in many other European countries because, as I noted earlier, women's life expectancy, though significantly above men's, does not compare very favourably with our European counterparts. The gender difference in longevity is highlighted if we look at the proportions surviving to different ages using the same life table data from which life expectancy is measured. Calculations based on mortality levels for 1994–6 indicate that for the UK as a whole 88 per cent of women will survive to 65 years but only 81 per cent of men; the difference then increases even further, with 70 per cent of women surviving to 75 but only 56 per cent of men, and 40 per cent of women surviving to 85 and only 22 per cent of men (ONS 1998a: table 2.20). Gender differences in life expectancy have tended to receive rather less attention than class inequalities even though they are marginally larger. The gender difference in life expectancy at birth of 5.6 years compares with the male class difference of 5.2 years and the female class difference of 3.4 years. This lack of attention may be because the gender difference is assumed, mistakenly, to be primarily biological and consequently unchangeable—a position I discuss and assess critically in Chapter 3. The gender difference in longevity is very considerable and should be a matter of concern.

The full extent of the current age-related gender differences can be seen if we compare the age-specific death rates given in Table 1.3. Table 1.11 presents the male–female ratio of these death rates and shows that the gender difference is now at its highest in the 15–24 age group—a period when deaths rates are generally very low and deaths from accidents and violence are very important as causes of death. At this stage in life men's death rates are currently around two and a half times as high as women's.

There are also marked gender differences in late middle age, when coronary heart disease leads to more deaths in men than women (this applies to all social classes). Indeed, it is the failure to cut back premature deaths in middle-aged men from coronary heart disease that makes so much difference to men's overall life expectancy (though male death rates from coronary heart disease have been declining).[22] This is a major problem for men, but also for their partners, since women (who anyway tend to be younger than their partners) frequently end up on their own in old age and are quite frequently impoverished—not least because their pensions are lower than men's (Arber and Ginn 1991: ch. 6). If men's longevity could match women's, this would make a radical change to the lives of both men and women and would increase the life expectancy of society as a whole.

In fact the situation in relation to gender is more complex than with social class, since in the case of class, as with age, the morbidity data are in line with mortality, the two both increasing as you move down the social scale. In the case of gender, men's higher levels of mortality are not matched by higher levels of reported sickness or greater use of health services (also often treated as a measure of morbidity); and using some measures we find the inverse

Table 1.11 Ratio of male to female age-specific death rates, 1931–1987, England and Wales

	0	1–4	5–14	15–24	25–34	35–44	45–54	55–64	65–74	75+
1931	1.36	1.14	1.09	1.05	1.27	1.30	1.39	1.35	1.33	1.15
1951	1.32	1.15	1.49	1.48	1.23	1.27	1.61	1.85	1.60	1.25
1971	1.31	1.19	1.53	2.19	1.60	1.48	1.64	2.00	1.97	1.36
1987	1.32	1.00	1.00	2.66	1.80	1.55	1.56	1.76	1.81	1.33

Source: Calculated from data in Illsley et al. (1991; table A4)

association between mortality and morbidity more typical of long-term trends.

The data on gender and morbidity are themselves not straightforward. Most studies indicate women use medical services more than men. The 1996 GHS figures show 19 per cent of women visiting a GP in the two weeks prior to interview, and only 13 per cent of men (ONS 1998c: table 8.20). However it is not clear that this results from higher morbidity. The extent of the gender difference varies with age, and almost all of women's greater use can be accounted for either by the need for contact with GPs in relation to reproduction or by gender differences in contact in relation to psychological health—issues examined more fully in Chapter 3. The data on in-patient stays in the twelve months prior to interview again show more women than men with in-patient stays (10 per cent as against 7 per cent), but this difference is accounted for by the greater number of stays amongst women aged 16–44 and 'is probably due to maternity stays' (ONS 1998c: 106). At other ages male rates for in-patient stays were marginally higher than female (ONS 1998c: table 8.32).

The data on reported sickness from the GHS in Table 1.4 show somewhat higher levels of limiting long-standing sickness and restricted activity in women than men, but no difference in the level of long-standing illness. If we take account of the difference in age distribution between men and women due to higher female longevity, which affects the male and female lifetime averages, the gender differences are very small, and in the case of long-standing illness, allowing for the difference in the age distribution actually generates a marginally higher figure for men than women. However, apart from mental health, there are other areas where women appear disadvantaged: one is mobility in later life. Arber and Ginn analysed the GHS data on reported capacity to do three things: walk down the road, get up and down stairs, and get around the house, and found that for most activities women in most five-year age bands from 65 and onwards were around twice as likely as men to report being unable to do them (1991: 113). In interpreting such data we need to remember that men's higher mortality means, other things being equal, that men who survive are a more selected group who are likely to be constitutionally fitter; in contrast, more women survive and so more are likely to develop chronic problems or incapacities (Manton 1982).

Taken together the data indicate, contrary to the claims of many, rather small gender differences in levels of morbidity as measured either by use of health services or in self-reported illness across the life span, with the exception of mental health and some disabilities in later life. However, this still leaves us with a conundrum: we might expect that, as with other cross-sectional data on health, men's higher mortality would be matched by higher morbidity, but this is not the case. We still, therefore, have to consider the possibility that the lack of concordance is due, as with the long-term trends, to the application of rather different illness thresholds. Alternatively, it may be that gender is an exception to the usual positive association between mortality and morbidity in cross-sectional data, and that applying the same illness thresholds to both men and women, women do actually have as much illness as men during their lives even though measured in terms of longevity they are healthier (the issue is considered more fully in Chapter 3).

Ethnicity

Data on mortality and morbidity in Britain by ethnicity also reveal important health inequalities. However the data are somewhat limited. *Our Healthier Nation* includes data on infant mortality by country of birth—a rather poor measure of ethnicity, but the only ethnic information available from death certificates. The infant mortality rate for those born in the UK and India was 6.2 per 1,000 live births for 1994–6; it was 5.9 for women born in East Africa, 6.3 for those born in Bangladesh, but 10.8 for those born in Pakistan and 11.2 for those born in the Caribbean (Secretary of State for Health 1998a: Fig. 3). A comparison with data from the mid-1970s shows that the raised infant mortality of those born in Pakistan or the Caribbean has persisted over the same period, though at that time those born in Pakistan had the highest infant mortality rates (Andrews and Jewson 1993).

There is also some comparative information on male death rates from coronary heart disease and strokes. Men born in West Africa and the Caribbean have lower death rates for coronary heart disease than the total population, whereas men born in South Asia, East Africa, Ireland, and Scotland have higher rates than the UK average. In contrast, those born in West Africa and the Caribbean have higher death rates from strokes than the UK average, but so, to a lesser extent, do those from South Asia, Scotland, Ireland, and East Africa (Wild and McKelgue, in Secretary of State for Health 1998a: 25).

Data on morbidity do not have to rely on country of birth for the measure of ethnicity, but usually group individuals according to the ethnic identity selected by the respondent. Studies show variations that correspond to the data on mortality. For example, a study carried out under the auspices of the Health Education Authority (1994) compared the self-reported health of four different minority ethnic groups, standardizing them for age and gender and comparing them with data for the UK population as a whole. The results are given in Table 1.12, and show that all the ethnic minority groups report, on average, poorer health than the population as a whole. Cultural differences in boundaries and thresholds of health may have influenced the responses, but it is interesting to note that the data are in line with the figures on infant

Table 1.12 Perceived health status by ethnic minority group

Health status	Afro-Caribbean	Indian	Pakistan	Bangladeshi	UK population
Very good	39	45	38	34	47
Fairly good	44	39	43	36	45
Fairly poor	9	11	14	20	6
Very poor	8	5	6	10	2

Source: Health Education Authority (1994: table 19)

mortality for the Caribbean and Pakistan minorities (though not for Bangladeshis).

The picture presented by the Health Education Survey on ethnic differences in morbidity is confirmed in a study by James Nazroo, *The Health of Britain's Ethnic Minorities* (1997a), which used data from the Fourth National Survey of Ethnic Minorities. The survey, which differentiated six ethnic minority groups, also relied on reports of health status from those interviewed. It showed that, in comparison with whites, some 29 per cent of whom described their health as only fair, poor, or very poor, these characterizations were employed by 32 per cent of those from ethnic minorities, with Caribbeans, Pakistanis, and Bangladeshis having the highest rates of self-assessed poor health with figures of 36, 36, and 38 per cent respectively. The figures for African, Asians, and Chinese, at 26 and 25 per cent respectively were below those for whites (Nazroo 1997a: 18). The survey also included data on a number of specific conditions such as diagnosed heart disease, hypertension, and diabetes, which again produced significant differences.

However, Nazroo contends that once adequate controls are introduced for social class many, though not all, of the identified differences in health disappeared. Here Nazroo differs from earlier commentators, who have tended to contend that the ethnic differences in health could not be accounted for by the differing class position of the ethnic groups (Marmot et al. 1984). Nazroo's argument is that it is not sufficient simply to look at the overall class position of the individual; it is also necessary to look at their location within a particular social class. He used a standard of living index based on overcrowding, access to amenities, and consumer durables to standardize the data for the different ethnic groups. Once this was accomplished, many of the differences in health were no longer statistically significant (Nazroo 1997a: ch. 5).

One area that merits special attention in relation to ethnic minority groups is that of mental health, and in particular the raised rates of admission for psychotic disorders amongst those from the Caribbean. These have been reported as between three and five times as high for whites in Britain (e.g. Harrison et al. 1988), with male rates especially high. However, a range of methodological weaknesses in many of these estimates have almost certainly invalidated the figures. For instance, until the 1991 Census it was difficult to estimate the size of the Afro-Caribbean population in Britain against which case data could be compared. A further concern has been the possibility of biases in the psychiatric assessments. The Fourth National Survey of Ethnic Minorities tried to deal with these methodological problems by using ethnically and language-matched interviews, follow-up interviews to validate the initial assessment, and age standardization, and showed rather smaller differences. The Caribbean rate of non-affective psychosis (primarily schizophrenia) was still a little over 50 per cent higher than for the white majority, but the difference was primarily due to raised female rates and was lower than in previous studies (Nazroo 1997b: table 3.6). The Irish had similarly raised rates (in this case due to higher male rates), whilst those for all other ethnic minority groups were lower than for whites. The Caribbean group also had higher levels of neurotic depression (but lower levels of anxiety) than whites, whilst the rates amongst all other ethnic groups except the Irish were lower than for whites (Nazroo 1997b: tables 3.3 and 3.4).

Conclusion

From the middle of the seventeenth century, when mortality levels started to decline, Britain has experienced a long-term improvement in the health of the population as measured in terms of life expectancy. With average life expectancy now over 74 years for men and over 79 years for women, and infant mortality now reduced to six deaths per 1,000 live births, there appears to be some cause for satisfaction. Nonetheless, there are grounds for serious disquiet at the overall picture. These come from three related sources. First, there are clear signs of the emergence or re-emergence of certain illnesses, including infections such as TB and AIDS and conditions such as asthma. Second, there are adverse trends in some of the important risk factors, most notably obesity, smoking amongst those aged 11–15, and exercise levels. And third, and most disturbingly of all, there are very marked class, gender, and ethnic inequalities in health within the population—inequalities that at one and the same time indicate the very poor levels of health of some members of the population and provide a measure of what could be achieved in terms of the overall health of the population. The task is not only to extend the life expectancy of men to match that of women, of the lowest social class to match that of the highest, or of certain ethnic minority groups to match that of the UK population as a whole, but to extend life expectancy by adding extra healthy years of life to the individual life span. This is the scale of the task that faces Britain.

Chapter 2

The Causes of Health and Illness

We can approach the task of explaining health and illness in a number of different ways. One contrast is between explanations that focus on biological processes versus those that focus on social processes. On the one hand, we can look at what goes on within the body and at bodily processes that either sustain health or generate illness—at the way in which certain nutrients improve resistance to disease, or the way in which a specific infectious micro-organism in the body leads to disease. On the other hand, we can look at which social processes make health or illness more likely—at how, for instance, poverty makes the consumption of an adequate diet much more difficult or at how patterns of sexual behaviour may affect the exposure to certain infectious micro-organisms. We might also add to this binary contrast between biological and social causes a set of psychological factors which may influence patterns of health and illness—for instance, feelings of loss and despair.

Another contrast in types of explanation of health and illness is between those focusing on heredity and those focusing on the environment: between genetic and environmental factors. This contrast has some analytic value, and the burgeoning area of genetics will have much to contribute to our understanding of health and illness. However, there is a tendency to see genes and environment as independent and to try to quantify the relative contribution of each, whereas in fact they are interdependent, and attempts to quantify their respective contribution are misconceived.[1]

Biological accounts of health and illness offer essentially complementary accounts to those emphasizing social and psychological factors, and genetic explanations are complementary to those that concentrate on environmental factors. However, for a variety of reasons biological processes are often treated as offering *the* explanation of health and illness and are given primacy over psychological and social processes, and the genetic is given primacy over the environmental. Historically, doctors have adopted very diverse, eclectic ideas about the causes of illness; yet with the development of the natural sciences they have increasingly paid most attention to biological processes in their accounts of the aetiology of disease and in the treatments they provide—a focus on biology which is currently manifest in a heavy concentration on research into genetic processes. Yet, as doctors themselves generally recognize, psychological, social, and environmental factors are also heavily implicated in the aetiology of diseases and can contribute to our understanding of health and illness. In particular they are very important to understanding some of the health inequalities described in the previous chapter, as well as to strategies for effective intervention. As a sociologist I want to focus on social and environmental factors as a counterbalance to medicine's customary biological focus, though biological and psychological processes will receive some attention, especially when considering the processes mediating between social factors and health and illness.

Discussions of the social causes of illness often make a contrast between material and cultural explanations. This was a key distinction in the discussion of the possible explanations of health inequalities in the influential *Black Report*. The contrast was between material inequalities associated with the distribution of resources, particularly poverty, which can have an impact on health, and on the other hand cultural or behavioural factors such as exercise, diet, and smoking (Townsend and Davidson 1988: ch. 6). In what follows I want to start with a fundamental contrast between *individual* and *societal* levels of analysis. This is a contrast between focusing on understanding health and illness at the level of the individual—an individual whose health is influenced by biological, psychological, and social processes—and focusing on the characteristics of the society or social groups in which people live their lives. To focus on the societal level of analysis is not the same as focusing on social factors at the individual level. For example, in focusing on social factors at the individual level I might look at whether a particular individual has sufficient resources to purchase an adequate diet, or at whether the individual is unemployed or not. At the societal level the concern would be with the way resources such as food are distributed across the population or with the pattern of unemployment or of social inequality.

Operating with this basic contrast between individual and societal levels, I make one further distinction at each level. At the individual level I distinguish between behaviour on the one hand and attributes and circumstances on the other; at the societal level I distinguish between the material environment mediated by the body and social relations mediated by subjectivity—a contrast that, as we shall see, differs from the material/cultural contrast more commonly deployed. At each level—individual and societal—the boundary between the two categories is not entirely precise; nonetheless analytically both distinctions are useful. These contrasts generate four types of approach to understanding the causes of health and illness. Type 1 involves a focus on individual behaviour; Type 2 concentrates on individual attributes and circumstances; Type 3 focuses on the material environment; and Type 4 concentrates on social relations. The four types are set out in Figure 2.1. I now examine each of the four types in turn.

Type 1 explanations: individual behaviour

A common type of approach in Western societies in both lay and professional circles to the task of explaining individual and group differences in levels and types of illness is in terms of individual 'health-related' behaviours. These are behaviours that have a generally well-established impact on the health of the individual by virtue of their impact on the body; they are sometimes termed 'risk' behaviours since the focus is usually on identifying behaviours that pose a

Figure 2.1 Types of explanatory approach

Individual level

Type 1: Behaviour
e.g. Smoking
Alcohol

Type 2: Attributes and circumstances
e.g. Genetic inheritance
Social class

Societal level

Type 3: Material environment and resource distribution
(mediated directly by the body)
e.g. Food supply
Air pollution
Poverty

Type 4: Social relations
(mediated by subjectivity)
e.g. Social cohesion
Employment relations

risk to health, and this formulation is increasingly fashionable, especially in the context of the discussion of the emergence of the so-called 'risk society' (see below).

The precise list of individual health-related behaviours that come under scrutiny varies, but ones frequently mentioned include behaviours such as diet, smoking, alcohol, illicit drugs, exercise, sexual relations, and, to a lesser extent, personal hygiene. In addition, a willingness or even desire to take risks can also be treated as a further factor that cuts across the risk behaviours so far mentioned and includes others such as a tendency to drive dangerously. The list changes over time as the perceived significance of specific behaviours changes. For example, a relatively recent addition to the list is sun-bathing, as the implications of prolonged exposure to the sun without protective creams have become apparent.[2] A range of strong empirical evidence typically underpins claims as to the dangers to health arising from these risk behaviours, although frequently there is considerable controversy about the precise boundaries and extent of the health risks. In the case of alcohol, for instance, evidence now indicates that moderate drinking may have benefits for health, though the adverse effects of sustained heavy drinking are well-established (Plant 1997).

These health-related behaviours have an impact on health and illness through the mediation of biological mechanisms. Two basic causal mechanisms can be distinguished. In some cases the health-related behaviour affects the individual's level of exposure to some 'noxious' agent, be it an infectious micro-organism, a chemical that is potentially harmful to the body, or some object that causes bodily injury. Under this basic mechanism it is useful to distinguish two possible pathways: the negative or 'pathogenic', through which illness is made more likely by increasing exposure to a micro-organism, and the positive or 'salutagenic' pathway, through which health is made more likely by reducing exposure to an infectious micro-organism (Antonovsky 1989). In other cases the health-related behaviour affects what can be broadly termed the body's general fitness and its consequent resistance to disease. Again, there are both negative and positive pathways: in the former the body's vulnerability to disease is increased; in the latter its resistance to illness is enhanced. The two basic biological mechanisms linking individual behaviour to health and illness with their respective negative and positive pathways are set out in Figure 2.2.

For example, particular patterns of sexual behaviour make the transmission of infectious micro-organisms such as hepatitis or herpes more likely, and in this case the causal mechanism follows Type 1(a). Smoking also operates according to Type 1(a), the noxious agent model, since it introduces chemicals into the body which affect lung and heart functioning. Both are instances of negative pathways. Personal hygiene also corresponds to Type 1(a) but is an instance of a positive pathway, since there is a reduced risk of exposure to noxious agents. In

Figure 2.2 Type 1 pathways linking individual behaviour to health and illness

1(a) Noxious agents

(i) Negative pathway

Individual behaviour → Increased exposure to noxious agents → Increased risk of illness

(ii) Positive pathway

Individual behaviour → Reduced exposure to noxious agents → Increased chance of health

1(b) Bodily vulnerability/resistance

(i) Negative pathway

Individual behaviour → Bodily vulnerability → Increased risk of illness

(ii) Positive pathway

Individual behaviour → Bodily resistance → Increased chance of health

the case of eating a healthy diet, the causal mechanism follows Type 1(b) with a positive pathway, since diet affects the nutritional status of the body, which has consequences for the resistance to infectious disease as well as for the maintenance of the healthy functioning of particular bodily organs such as the heart. Conversely, a diet with an insufficiency of certain key nutritional elements, such as vitamin C, would be a Type 1(b) negative pathway. Exercise acts to maintain healthy functioning of the heart and lungs and is a Type 1(b) positive pathway. Of course, the separation between Type 1(a) and Type1(b) pathways is introduced here for its analytic value. In practice it is the interaction between, say, the presence of an infectious micro-organism and bodily resistance/vulnerability that is crucial.

Behaviours placed in the category of 'health-related' are usually assumed to be the product of individual action and decision-making, and therefore matters over which the individual has some control and for which they can be held responsible, though the frequent use of the term 'lifestyle' in this context suggests that there is some social patterning to the behaviours and that cultural influences are at work. However, even when the idea of lifestyles is invoked—a concept that was originally intended to suggest the social and cultural context of individual behaviour (Coreil et al. 1994)—the implication is still that individuals have some choice over what they do and are free to adopt or reject a given lifestyle. It is accepted, of course, that not all individuals are equally motivated towards the maintenance of health, and not always equally knowledgeable about the health risks associated with particular behaviours. Some prefer to take risks with their health or do not realize they are taking risks, and as a result may fall into one of the 'high-risk' groups for a particular condition—smokers for lung cancer, overweight people for heart disease, and so forth.[3] From this point of view health can be enhanced in the population either by increasing knowledge of the health consequences of particular behaviours (though frequently individuals are already aware of the health dangers of their behaviour) or, more importantly, by increasing motivation (for instance, by making health a higher priority for the individual). Hence the proclaimed need for better health education which is designed to increase knowledge and improve motivation.

A focus on health-related behaviour is the type of explanatory account frequently adopted by government and policy-makers when they consider the possibility of any preventive intervention, and was particularly visible under Conservative administrations from 1979 to 1997. The 1992 *The Health of the Nation* White Paper (Secretary of State for Health 1992), for example, which set targets for reducing disease and improving health in relation to coronary heart disease and strokes, cancers, mental illness, accidents, and HIV/AIDS and sexual health, focused largely on changing individual behaviour. There are a number of reasons for the common bias towards individual behaviour. First, it is consistent with the individualism that characterizes much medical and clinical work, where the requirement is first and foremost to attend to the needs of the individual patient.[4] Second, it fits well with assumptions about human rationality and the capacity for self-control which have been very pervasive since the eighteenth century. Third, it relates to, and is arguably a reflection of, the concerns in late modern society about the development of self-identity and lifestyle through individual choice (see Giddens 1991: 5). And fourth, it avoids the sorts of interventions indicated by analyses at the societal level, interventions which often require more radical and more politically committed intervention. It is far easier politically to exhort individuals to stop smoking than to ban cigarette advertising, not least because of the vested interests of the tobacco industry as well as other industries that may benefit from cigarette advertising (the controversies surrounding the banning of cigarette advertising through sports sponsorship shows some of the problems). Equally, it is politically easier to encourage individuals to eat healthier foods than to regulate the very powerful and increasingly global food industry. Does this matter? Are there any fundamental objections to taking the politically easier route, or indeed to the whole focus on explaining illness in terms of individual behaviour?

There are two major, related problems concerning the dominant focus on health-related behaviours. First, and very importantly, it ignores the social and cultural context in which individual behaviour is located, which needs to be examined if we are to have a better understanding of the individual behaviour in question and, crucially, are to be able to intervene effectively if we want to change it. Individuals may choose to buy white bread made from refined flours rather than healthier brown bread, but this may be because white bread is cheaper than brown and this is the type of bread they are used to and therefore like. What is needed in this case is an analysis that looks both at the way bread is produced, at the way bread prices are set and at the marketing of bread which may shape individual preferences, and at the distribution of income within the society. All these factors may underpin an individual's decision to buy white rather than brown bread. It is for this reason that health education activities which focus at the individual level are so often ineffective.

Second, and equally importantly, some of the factors influencing the individual's health or that of a population cannot properly be said to be mediated by individual behaviour. There is a whole set of determinants of health that cannot be captured through a focus on health-related behaviours, even if they are placed in their social and cultural context. Consider, for example, the consumption by individuals of contaminated food or water, such as beef contaminated by BSE, milk contaminated by nuclear radiation, or water contaminated by industrial effluents. It is theoretically possible, of course, to talk of the consumption of these substances as a matter of individual, health-related behaviour. Certainly individuals eat the food or drink the water in question, but to call these health-related behaviours is absurd and inappropriate since, as we have seen, the term 'health-related behaviour' implies that individuals have some choice in the situation and some control over what they do. If individuals have no knowledge of the contamination, or have no choice of alternative sources of non-contaminated food or water, then to talk of health-related behaviours would be misguided. It would be naive to suggest to a woman living in the Ukraine in an area where water and milk are contaminated from nuclear radiation, an area to which she is tied by family and work, that she can choose a healthier lifestyle, or that people in Wales and Scotland whose land and cattle were exposed to nuclear radiation following Chernobyl could do very much as individuals to reduce their risks of ill-health. Certainly, once the risks of BSE were made known to a wider public, the avoidance of beef products in one's diet could reasonably begin to be described as a health-related behaviour since there are dietary alternatives (though given the limited information required by law, identifying all products with some substance derived from beef can be very difficult). But prior to this individuals had no knowledge of the consequences and could not take action to reduce their risks of ill-health. Moreover, even now it is hard for the public to determine the risks of eating, say, British beef, since even academic scientists do not agree on the risks involved.

Some attempts have been made to assess the relative significance of individual health-related behaviours to health. Wilkinson (1996: 63–6), refers to a study carried out by Marmot and his colleagues (1978) of coronary heart disease amongst civil servants—a disease where a number of identifiable health-related behaviours are known to be involved, such as smoking, diet, and lack of exercise. He argues that even for this condition at best some 40 per cent of the observed difference could be accounted for by four risk factors—blood pressure, cholesterol, smoking, and height—leaving 60 per cent to be accounted for by other factors. However Marmot and his co-workers themselves qualify this claim by noting that it is dependent on their particular set of health-related factors (they also included blood glucose, body mass, and reported physical activity, but these had little impact) and on the ways in which they were measured. Moreover, it needs to be noted that the Marmot study was a study of risk *factors*, not just risk *behaviours*, and included a mixture of health-related behaviours—smoking and exercise—and of individual attributes, some of which are arguably outcomes of health-related behaviours—body mass and possibly cholesterol and blood pressure, and some such as height less directly related to the individual's health behaviour. Other studies have also questioned the importance of individual behaviour to health. The Health and Lifestyle Survey (Blaxter 1990), which paid considerable attention to health-related behaviours, found their importance depended on social circumstances. They were significant amongst the middle classes, whose social circumstances were generally favourable; they were of much less importance in the working-class groups, where social conditions exerted far more influence. As this particular finding suggests, it needs to be remembered that the importance of selected individual behaviours, as against other factors operating at the individual level such as socio-economic circumstances or indeed genetic differences, will vary across time and place, as well as depending on what is placed in the category of individual behaviour. For example, to the extent that socio-economic circumstances are uniform across the individuals or groups in question then individual behaviours will become more important in accounting for differences in health.[5] Where socio-economic circumstances are highly differentiated they are likely to be more important in accounting for variations in health than individual behaviours.

Individual behaviours do therefore need to be part of the analysis. However, it is also vital to extend the analysis to social circumstances. This needs to be done in two rather different ways. First, at the individual level we need to consider all the other factors that influence an individual's health apart from their individual behaviour, including their social circumstances, but also what I have chosen to call their attributes. And second, we need to place both their individual behaviour and their attributes and circumstances into the context of the social and economic organization of society—that is, to move from the individual to the societal level. I want next to consider accounts of health and illness that focus on individual-level attributes and social circumstances.

Type 2 explanations: individual-level attributes and circumstances

A focus on individual-level attributes and circumstances is particularly associated with the epidemiological approach to the study of health and illness. Epidemiology is the study of the distribution of diseases across populations, and is first and foremost an empirical, methodological approach in which comparisons are made between the health and illness of groups or individuals differentiated by certain characteristics. In the classic epidemiological studies of cholera, Dr John Snow, who believed that cholera resulted from an infectious organism spread by polluted water, established in a study in 1854 that those who obtained water from the Southall and Vauxhall water company were more likely to develop cholera because the water was contaminated by the organism; those supplied by a different pump were far less likely to develop the disease. In fact Snow's aetiological account can be used to draw attention either to the societal or to the individual level. We can either focus on the adequacy of water supplies in particular areas of London (or elsewhere) or we can treat geographical location (and hence the source of their water supply) as an individual attribute or circumstance which affects the individual's chances of developing cholera, the causal pathway involving both social and biological processes. Epidemiology does not therefore necessarily require us to focus on the individual level. However, since much of the work proceeds by the establishment of correlations between patterns of morbidity and mortality and certain social characteristics of individuals, it is often oriented to the individual level and can and does embrace individual behaviour such as smoking, as well as individual attributes and circumstances such as where someone lives and the water supply they receive.[6]

The domain of factors that can be studied at the individual level and treated as individual attributes or circumstances is very extensive, and together with individual behaviour can constitute an exhaustive list of individual-level influences on health. On the one hand, there is the full range of social attributes and circumstances that are commonly used to characterize and map individuals—

sometimes called 'face-sheet' variables—including the individual's age, gender, marital status, social class, ethnicity, education, income, employment status, region, etc. Most of these can have a profound impact on a person's chances of health and illness, and those with the most marked impact are often now termed 'risk factors'. Consider, for example, age. As I noted in the previous chapter, patterns of health and illness are highly dependent on age, though the precise relation with age varies across time and place (the phase of the epidemiological transition is important). Whilst infants are especially vulnerable to disease, particularly where infectious illnesses are common, in later childhood and early adulthood disease and death become rarer, only to increase again at later ages (precisely when depends on the society). Marital status is also important, with the married generally having better health than the divorced, widowed, or single—a contrast that is usually more marked for men, who appear to gain more from marriage. On the other hand, there are individual biological and psychological characteristics, such as height (one of the Marmot risk factors that, as I noted in Chapter 1, is positively associated with health), weight, and temperament which also affect health and illness.

These diverse, individual-level attributes and circumstances are underpinned both by genetic and environmental factors and by biological and social processes. Age, for instance, is not simply a biological fact, it is also a social category governed by social expectations. Gender is in part a genetic given but is also socially shaped and transformed (the term 'sex' highlights its biological significance, 'gender' the social shaping).

Given this diverse domain of individual-level attributes and circumstances, it is not surprising to find that the causal mechanisms linking them to health or illness are also diverse. They include biological mediation via noxious agents as, for instance, when by virtue of where they live an individual is exposed to such an agent, as well as mediation by biological vulnerability and resistance as when, for example, by virtue of when and where someone lives their diet is very restricted. Genetic factors, for example, often operate by increasing or decreasing an individual's biological vulnerability to certain environmental factors. In some cases their genetic inheritance is such that illness is likely: an example would be those who inherit the gene for Huntingdon's chorea— a progressive degenerative disease of the brain which typically emerges in middle age. More commonly, the outcome of the genetic inheritance depends on the presence or absence of certain environmental conditions and the situation is one of a complex interaction of causes.

Individual-level attributes are also linked to health and illness via the mediation of psychological mechanisms, and the contrast between bodily and psychological mediation is fundamental to my distinction at the societal level between the material environment and social relations. The best-known and most widely studied of these is stress (see e.g. Totman 1990; Elstad 1998). 'Stress' is a term commonly used to link social circumstances to a variety of outcomes including ill-health (but also to various types of deviance including violent behaviour and poor performance at work), the precise usage varying from context to context. An important distinction is between its use to characterize the situation a person is in (where the terms 'stressful' or 'stressor' make it clear that it is the situation itself which is being described) and its use to characterize the individual's response to that situation—the stress reaction or stressful experience. In discussing the psychological mediation between individual-level factors and health and illness the circumstances (for instance, unemployment or being widowed) are the stressors and the experience of stress—the reaction—the mediating mechanism.

Stress as a reaction has two dimensions: psychological and physical; at the psychological level, the individual is likely to feel tense, anxious, fearful or distressed, at the physical level there will be changes to adrenalin levels, heart rate, and so forth. It is these physical changes associated with the psychological state of stress that make ill-health more likely, especially if the stress is chronic—that is, the stressful situation is ongoing and the person continues to experience stress as a result. There is clear evidence, for instance, that chronic stress affects the immune system and consequently resistance to disease (Totman 1990: ch. 5).

Precisely how we can best measure the levels of stress individuals encounter is hotly contested. Some use standard measures of stress, in which weights are attached to a fixed set of events or situations (such as divorce or unemployment) in terms of how stressful they are to most people and then calculate, using a fixed set of questions, the total level of stress the individual faces.[7] Others argue that we need to look at the significance of particular circumstances for the individual in question in order to get an accurate measure of the level of stress to which they are exposed (they may want to get divorced, or have hated their job), though this can make it difficult to differentiate the level of stress to which someone is exposed from their reaction to it.[8]

Whilst these are important methodological debates, they do not call into question the substantial body of evidence that indicates that when faced with stressful situations individuals are more likely to become ill either physically or mentally. A number of studies have, for instance, shown that those who are widowed, especially men, are much more likely to die during the following six months in comparison with control groups (Bowling 1987). We might say in everyday terms that they have lost the will to live. Or we could say that they found the loss of their spouse highly stressful and this psychological stress made death more likely, perhaps leading them to suicide or, by its impact on the immune system, reducing their resistance to illness. Other studies have shown that the incidence of coronary heart disease is more likely in situations of stress (Cooper et al. 1985). In addition there is a range of 'psychosomatic diseases' where the psychological element is so widely accepted that this is not only built into the categorization of the disorder but informs routine discussions of the condition in both lay and medical contexts: stomach ulcers is one such condition. Stress had also been shown to be a cause of some psychiatric disorders, especially the neuroses (Brown and Harris 1989). There is also evidence of links between unemployment, stress, and illness which are discussed more fully in Chapter 3.

However, just as we need to consider the body's resistance to illness as well as the presence or absence of noxious agents, we also need to consider psychological resistance and vulnerability in the face of stress. George Brown and Tirril Harris's classic study, *Social Origins of Depression* (1978), provided evidence that when women (no men were included in the study) faced stressful events or ongoing difficulties the likelihood of becoming depressed depended on four vulnerability factors: the lack of an intimate, confiding relationship, the presence of three or more children in the home, the loss of their mother before the age of 11, and whether or not they had paid work outside the home.[9] They were given the status of vulnerability factors because the data indicated that they only made depression more likely in the presence of stressful events or difficulties. The interaction between the four factors was complex and the first was the most important. The authors noted that the obverse of vulnerability is 'coping' and that those with an intimate, confiding relationship—now usually described in the literature as one form of 'social support'—were better able to cope with the stresses they faced: a finding repeated in numerous other studies (Brugha 1995).

The different pathways linking individual attributes and circumstances to health and illness are set out in Figure 2.3. which combines the pathogenic and salutagenic models. The first two types involve bodily, the second two psychological mediation. However, individual attributes and circumstances, like individual behaviour, need to be placed in their societal context. This is essential if we are to have a better understanding of the health inequalities outlined in the first chapter, and if we are to be able to produce appropriate and effective health policies.

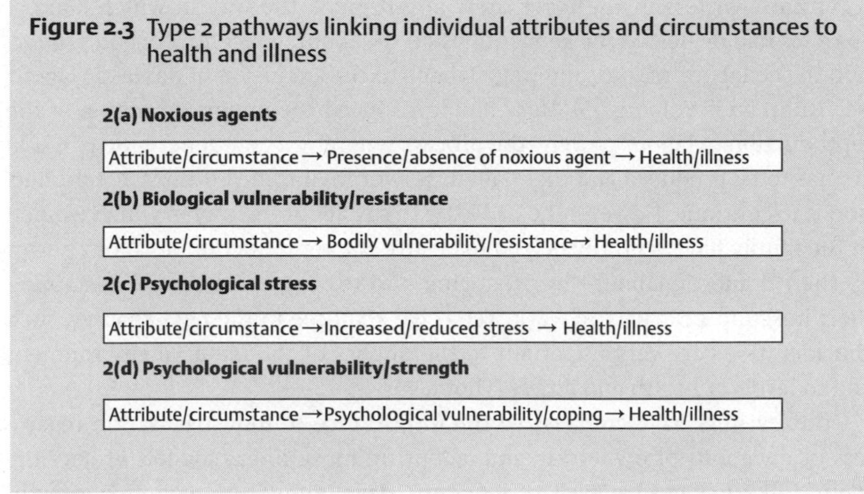

Figure 2.3 Type 2 pathways linking individual attributes and circumstances to health and illness

Type 3 explanations: the material environment and resource distribution

There can be no doubt that individuals' health-related behaviour and their attributes and circumstances, which influence patterns of health and illness, are shaped by their material environment at the societal level and by the way resources are distributed within the society—a material environment and patterns of resource distribution that result from the political and economic organization of society.

There have been various attempts to characterize the differences in political and economic organization of societies. Marx's focus on differing modes of production—fundamental distinctions in the way economic activity is organized, with a key contrast between communist and capitalist societies, based on the pattern of ownership of the means of production—has been highly influential. Since this binary division permits only limited differentiation between societies it has been common, for instance, to distinguish between either types or stages of capitalism, as in descriptions such as *laissez-faire*, monopoly, managed, state, or 'disorganized' capitalism, or early, proto-, advanced and late capitalism. Whatever the differentiation, the way in which productive activity is organized is seen as fundamental to the character of society and the basis of social divisions within it as are concepts such as power and interest. Whilst many of Marx's predictions have not been realized, his attention to production, wage labour, social divisions, power, and interests are still crucial to any adequate analysis of the economic and social organization of society.

Feminist writers in the 1970s drew attention to the way in which Marxist analyses had neglected the gender division of labour, concentrating on production in the labour market and wage labour to the exclusion of domestic labour (see Kuhn and Wolpe 1978). Marx had introduced the important notion of the reproduction of labour power—the process whereby a new generation of workers has to be produced and their labour power maintained if capitalist production is to continue. However, he had little to say about the way in which women in the family have typically helped to ensure the reproduction of labour power by their domestic labour—by producing and rearing children and sustaining their husband's capacity to work. Yet as we shall see in the next chapter, such considerations are very important to the quality of the material environment and to levels of health and illness (Thomas 1995).

Other writers have emphasized the importance of industrialisation regardless of questions of ownership and, adopting more linear models of development, talk of stages or levels of economic development or economic growth, often measured in terms of the average per capita income of a society. Some focus on the crucial importance of shifts between an economy dominated by agricultural activity to one dominated by industrial production; others focus on the shifting balance between primary, secondary, and tertiary production. Yet others think in terms of modernization—a term that tries to capture both economic and cultural change, often differentiating stages of modernization, with terms such as 'early modern', 'modern', and 'late' or 'post-modern' society. Here, particularly amongst those who talk of the emergence of post-modern societies or of late modernity, the emphasis often shifts from production to consumption, which is, for instance, seen as crucial to the social divisions within advanced Western societies as they enter the twenty-first century.

We cannot, of course, settle the highly contested theoretical and empirical debates about characterizing and differentiating societies here. What is crucial is the fundamental importance attributed by many of these theorists to the political and economic organization of society and to the distribution of resources—an importance that can be applied to the understanding of patterns of health and illness. In order to examine their importance to health and illness, I want to consider three aspects of the material environment which have particular relevance to health and are shaped by, and part of, the political and economic organization of society and of resource distribution, including the conditions of wage and domestic labour. The three are the production of food, the supply of water, and the regulation of atmospheric pollution. All relate to basic biological necessities for healthy human existence: food, water and air. I also consider a fourth aspect of the material environment: protection from accident and injury. All also need to be examined in the context of aspects of

Figure 2.4 Type 3 explanations of illness: the material environment

Environment →	Behaviours/attributes/ circumstances →	Noxious agent/ bodily vulnerability →	Health/illness

the political and economic organization of society and the distribution of resources, including production and wage and domestic labour.

At the individual level, the four features influence health and illness as attributes, circumstances, or behaviours whose impact is mediated either by noxious agents or by bodily resistance and vulnerability. Indeed, one of the defining characteristics of the material environment as it is analysed here is that it operates directly on the body and does not involve psychological mediation in its impact on health and illness (the material environment is, of course, itself a product of human action and human culture).

The Type 3 explanation of illness is set out in Figure 2.4; at the individual level it may involve behaviours, attributes, or circumstances.

The production of food

Food is vital to the health of any group of individuals, since those who are malnourished—either because they do not have sufficient food overall, or because they do not have a diet adequate in certain nutrients—are more susceptible to illness and disease. A diet needs to include sufficient calories, but also sufficient proteins and vitamins. Food also needs to be free from contamination either from infectious micro-organisms or from other noxious substances such as chemicals. Furthermore, diets should not be excessive, and particular substances, harmless or even beneficial in small quantities, may be dangerous in excess—alcohol is but one example.

The nutritional adequacy of diets is particularly pertinent to a population's resistance to infectious disease. Those who are malnourished are more likely to fall ill, to have more serious illness, and to take more time to recover if they do, whereas those who are well nourished have a greater resistance to disease. A review by Newberne and Williams on the effects of nutrition on the course of infections concluded:

> Grossly inadequate intakes of protein and other specific nutrients are today resulting in extreme degrees of malnutrition and concomitant infectious disease. It seems likely that the interaction between nutrition and infection are more important in animal and

human populations than one would predict from the results of laboratory investigations. It must be remembered that the interaction between nutrition and infection is dynamic, being frequently characterised by synergism and less commonly, by antagonism, and that control of malnutrition and infection are interdependent, so that the course of a disease is intimately related to the nutritional status of the host. (quoted in McKeown 1976: 134)

A World Health Organization report in 1973 concluded: 'For the time being an adequate diet is the most effective "vaccine" against most of the diarrhoeal, respiratory and other common infections' (quoted in McKeown 1976: 136).

In advanced industrial societies calorific intakes are usually adequate, and gross malnutrition is relatively uncommon, but diets may not contain all the desirable nutrients, or may be either excessive in quantity or unbalanced, leading to obesity or an excess of certain substances, such as fats. It is becoming increasingly clear, for example, that the immune system is affected by the presence of various nutrients and that, for instance, certain nutrients increase protection against cancer via the immune system. Equally, food needs to be free from significant contaminants. Recent examples of food contamination include BSE in beef, which was linked to a shift in the food fed to cattle from plants to a high protein animal diet in order to hasten development and to changes in the processing of that food, as well as salmonella in dairy products such as eggs and chicken, linked to the highly intensive battery farm production of chickens. There is also growing concern about the effect of pesticide residues such as organo-phosphates on plants, and about the evidence indicating that the routine use of antibiotics in animal husbandry is increasing the development and spread of bacteria resistant to antibiotics. And there is now serious concern about the possible impact of genetic engineering on crops. Genetically modified crops are currently being grown in Britain on a trial basis in conditions which do not fully protect against the possibility of cross-pollination with other crops. Moreover, the labelling of foods is inadequate: recent studies indicate that it is not possible for the consumer to identify which food stuffs contain genetically modified ingredients.

The capacity to supply adequate food, including the necessary nutrients, to all members of the population without contamination is a major task of society, and the ways it does so reflects its economic organization. In less developed societies the importance of food to the survival of the group was widely recognized, and securing food was a major focus of human activity as in hunter gatherer and peasant societies, where populations were vulnerable to droughts, poor harvests, and the destruction of plants or animals, and famines were not infrequent. Urbanization and industrialization meant major changes in the production and distribution of food, with a far higher proportion being produced commercially for sale on the market and the industrialization of food production. This had important advantages, since it generally increased food supplies and in the long run often meant lower food prices. However, it also meant that the quality and type of food was in the hands of large-scale landowners and food companies who could pursue their own interests rather than those of the consumers (for instance, sacrificing quality to profits). It also meant that individuals were dependent on their family's wages for the possibility of obtaining food. With the high levels of income inequality common in industrial capitalist societies, some families faced and still face considerable difficulty in securing adequate food for all members (an issue discussed more fully in Chapter 3, where the distribution of food within families is also considered). Estimates suggest that even at the end of the nineteenth century some 30 per cent of the population were malnourished (Blane 1987).

The contamination and adulteration of food, as well as the destruction of nutrients, is always a major threat, and the quality of food bears no linear relationship to the level of economic development of a society. New technologies may reduce production costs but do not necessarily improve quality. An obvious example in Britain is the development in the 1950s of the Chorleywood method of producing bread by large-scale flour millers, who were taking over bread production (David 1977). This method modified the period of time taken to mature dough by using mechanical agitation in high-speed mixers. It allowed greater use of low-protein English wheat (saving on import costs) and increased the absorption of larger quantities of water into highly refined flours (generally the more refined the flour the greater the absorption of water), so reducing costs and increasing profits, as well as increasing the use of chemical bleaches (bleached flour was more suitable for the new machinery). The result was a revolution in bread production and consumption, with a shift to widespread use of white bread made from less nutritious flour rather than the healthier brown bread—an example of the importance of material environment rather than individual health-related behaviour, since it was the industry that produced the change in the pattern of consumption because the price for the new Chorleywood bread was considerably lower. This increased demand, and though customers benefited from lower prices, they did not benefit in terms of quality.

Marketing also plays an important role in patterns of food consumption and is widely used by food companies to generate demand for their products in the pursuit of higher profits and an expanding market. A classic example has been the creation of demand for cow's milk products for babies as an alternative to breast milk that goes well beyond the necessary use of cow's milk when mothers are unable to feed their own babies. This is a problem because breast milk has been shown to be better for babies, as it increases immunity to disease. Recent scandals in this area have tended to focus on the sale and marketing of these products in Third World countries, yet there are also areas for concern in countries like Britain. Only around two-thirds of babies in Britain are now breast-fed in the first month and after four months the percentage is only 27 per cent, some of the lowest figures in Europe.

Many of the food companies are now international in their operations and there has been an increasing globalization of food production and marketing over recent years. Since the final decades of the nineteenth century Britain has relied heavily on imports for its food; with the entry into the European Community much of its trade in food is with Europe, and many of the key companies are global. These companies shape what people eat in a variety of ways. They influence patterns of consumption across the population not only by advertising and marketing but also by the prices they charge, with price especially important for low-income families. They also influence consumption by the ways in which they conserve and preserve food (including the use of various additives that increase shelf life) and by the ingredients they use in their cooked and ready-to-use foods. This is increasingly important as more and more people rely on ready-prepared foods and the domestic labour of food preparation is reduced—a trend associated with increasing affluence, with higher proportions of women in paid jobs outside the home, and with more people living on their own. The recent controversies surrounding the use of genetically modified crops, and the nigh impossibility of determining whether a food you buy does contain such products, is a recent example of the difficulties facing the consumer and of the power of the food companies.

The power of the food industry and its increasing globalization poses considerable problems for governmental attempts at regulation. The extent to which the industry is adequately regulated varies enormously between countries and over time, although bodies such as the European Union are now playing an increasing role in food regulation. In Britain food regulation has been part of the business of the Ministry of Agriculture, Fisheries, and Food, which combined looking at the interests of food producers with those of protecting food consumers leading to considerable potential conflicts of interest. The Labour Government initially set out plans to introduce a new Food Standards Agency under the Department of Health independent of the Ministry of Agriculture, and after some delay the agency looks set to be established.[10] From the point of view of the population's health there can be little doubt of the desirability of achieving a clear separation of the regulation of the food industry, designed to protect consumers, from providing support for food producers and retailers, whose interests usually differ markedly from those of consumers, though national regulation is becoming less significant in the face of globalization of many aspects of the food industry. One of the major problems of regulation, however, is the danger of regulatory capture (Bernstein 1955): that regulators, even if carefully chosen as independent, can be captured by the industry that is being regulated, coming to share its ideas and perspectives, though in some cases regulators may be able to resist these pressures (Abraham 1995: 23–4).

The supply of water

Water is essential to health in three important ways. First, water for individual consumption is necessary for the survival of the human body; without it, or in situations of water scarcity, the individual will die or their resistance to illness will be weakened. Second, water when contaminated either by infectious micro-organisms or by noxious substances such as certain chemicals directly exposes the individual to the risk of illness. Third, access to an adequate supply of clean water is important to bodily cleanliness, including adequate sanitation, and the maintenance of clean, healthy living and working environments free of contaminants.

The range of infectious diseases transmitted through water includes cholera, typhoid fever, and amoebic dysentery as well as Weil's disease (the infectious micro-organism can be excreted into water by rats). Lead, commonly used in piping in the Victorian era, leaches into water and has a deleterious effect on brain growth, whilst arsenic and nuclear residues are other water pollutants that pose a threat to health.

Like food, the provision of adequate water supplies is a major task for society and cannot simply be viewed as an individual responsibility. Again, the problems posed by urbanization and industrialization for the supply of water were enormous because of the concentrations of people they engendered, as well as the new and ever-expanding demands for water for industrial and domestic purposes. Severe droughts can cause enormous problems, as can the lack of adequate sanitation leading to the contamination of water. Historically, faecal contamination of water arising from human or animal excrement has been the overriding problem with water supplies. In advanced industrial societies like Britain this type of contamination of water supplies has been reduced, but there are still major problems concerning the discharge of sewage from the sea, and a high percentage of beaches do not meet European standards of cleanliness. Contamination from industrial effluents is also still a significant problem.

In Britain, improvements in sanitation were a major focus of public health activity in the nineteenth century and helped to reduce the faecal contamination of water, although even by the middle of this century some houses still did not have hot water (see Chapter 3). There was, however, little control of industrial effluents, including poisons such as arsenic. The discharge of industrial substances into rivers was seen as the price that had to be paid for industrial progress. The Royal Commission on River Pollution in 1867 described how the River Lea was blackened with industrial wastes:

> Large quantities of various metallic salts, dye-stuffs, brimstone, and other objectionable, and, in some cases, poisonous materials are, after use in the processes of cleansing, bleaching, and dyeing of the goods, discharged into the stream from which water for the domestic use of a large portion of London is drawn. (quoted in Wohl 1983: 234)

Much of this obvious industrial pollution has now been controlled, but there are still important instances of illegal pollution (and often relatively small fines if a case goes to court). Moreover, some of the pollution is not necessarily illegal. An important example is nitrates. These are widely used in large-scale farming to increase crop yields. But they inevitably spread into the soil, and through the soil they get into underground waters and into the water system. Ingested nitrates are converted into nitrites which have carcinogenic properties. The control of this practice requires, however, greater regulation of the activities of farmers than has currently been accepted. Contamination of water, including sea water, by nuclear residues also occurs through various discharges, and these residues can get into the food chain.

The privatization of the water industry has arguably made regulation more difficult. For example, it has recently been noted that the number of rats in Britain's sewage system has increased, and the water companies are more reluctant to play their part in controlling them. A further related problem has been the decimation of local government over the past twenty years, since it was the local authorities who played a crucial role in controlling water pollution and in sanitation, although local authorities still employ environmental health officers. Privatization has also increased concerns about the cost of water and the cutting off of water supplies to those who do not pay their bills because of financial problems. The use of pre-paid water meters, with companies then permitted to cut off supplies without seeking authorization, has been a recent source of controversy.

The issue is not, however, only one of ensuring good-quality water, it is also one of sufficiency. Ironically, some of the very measures which improve sanitation and facilitate greater cleanliness in work and domestic environments, as well as reducing the labour, largely domestic, involved in keeping clean, at the same time increase the demand for water. Water closets, sinks, showers, baths, and washing-machines in the home all push up demand, as do similar workplace facilities. This makes the task of ensuring an adequate supply of water more and more difficult, and on a global level it is increasingly argued that control over water supplies is likely to prove a major source of international conflict. In Britain, one problem which is not being tackled fully is the limitations of the existing infrastructure for supplying water and sewage. Much of the infrastructure was laid down in the Victorian era and needs replacing. Consequently there are numerous leaks of sewage which have public health consequences, as well as significant losses of water through seepage. Considerable investment in water pipes and drainage is needed to replace the infrastructure, and policies need to be developed to curtail the usage of water whilst ensuring clean, hygienic environments.

Air pollution

Clean air to breathe is also vital to health. Like food and water, air can be contaminated by infectious micro-organisms or noxious agents, or may lack elements essential to health, most obviously sufficient oxygen. Some (though not excessive) exposure to sunlight is also beneficial to health. Airborne infectious diseases include diseases where there is direct transmission of micro-organisms from one person to another through droplets or droplet nuclei or indirectly by dust particles which may fall on bedding, floors, and clothes. These include diphtheria, whooping cough, measles, and chickenpox. Airborne contaminants include various substances which have an adverse effect on the respiratory system, again often associated with industrial processes broadly defined. Classic instances are the diseases associated with mining where miners have to work in a closely confined space, where the atmosphere is polluted, and there is a lack of fresh air. Respiratory problems amongst miners have been a major source of illness and disease and include conditions such as emphysema and silicosis. More recent examples include asbestosis, generated by exposure to asbestos which proved to be highly carcinogenic. Indeed, paid work, particularly in mining and manufacturing, has been a major source of exposure to atmospheric pollutants—an issue examined more fully in the next chapter. Overcrowding in domestic environments also increases the chances of the airborne spread of noxious agents, including infectious micro-organisms; and chemical pollutants picked up in the workplace may be spread to domestic environments. For instance, asbestos may cling to clothes and affect women who wash them.

The availability of clean air is clearly not simply a matter of nature, but is a product of human activity. Industrial processes, if unregulated, pollute the air and pose an important threat to health. Again, throughout much of the nineteenth century atmospheric pollution generated by industry was hardly regulated in Britain, and the impact was not restricted to those engaged in paid labour in trade and manufacturing. Smoke from factories was allowed to rise into the air of cities and towns unchecked, blackening buildings and causing respiratory problems amongst the population who lived there. The term 'Black Country', applied to one of the industrial heartlands of Britain, signalled the high level of pollution caused by industry, as did the epithet 'the old smoke' used to describe London.

During the twentieth century the regulation of atmospheric pollution from factories has increased and the pollution from coal-burning, which was generated by domestic as well as factory consumption, has been reduced (the smogs disrupting London life in the early 1950s were one force for change). But other forms of air pollution have become important. Pollution from cars, which have become the dominant form of transport in the twentieth century, has replaced pollution from factories as a major threat to health. The consequences are various. Cars contaminate the air with pollutants that can directly affect health, for example through the emission of lead from petrol and particulates from diesel fuel. Cars are also implicated in the global warming that appears to be occurring, which is itself a threat to health, including from a reduction in the ozone layer which increases skin cancers.

Cigarette smoking constitutes another form of atmospheric pollution to which attention has been drawn in recent years. In addition to the health effects on the individual smoker, those who work or live alongside smokers face negative health consequences through 'passive smoking' since nicotine is released into the atmosphere and is inhaled by others. Recent estimates indicate that the health consequences of passive smoking are considerable. In countries like Britain there have been efforts to control smoking in some public places on public health grounds, including work environments, but there are still some public spaces where smoking is common, most obviously bars and pubs.

Protection from accidents and injury

A major way in which the material environment can affect the health of a population is through the extent to which it exposes individuals to accident and injury. A marked feature of the working conditions of wage labourers in early industrialization was the direct risks of accident and injury, often fatal, to which workers were exposed. The high death rates from accidents amongst miners in the nineteenth century are well known, and fatalities still occur even with much greater regulation (there is some evidence that the privatization of coal mining may have lead to an increase in the rate of fatal accidents in mines, though absolute numbers have fallen sharply along with the near collapse of coal mining in Britain over the last decade and a half). The levels of accidents and injury in factories in the nineteenth century were often high, with individuals frequently maimed or incapacitated by injury. Significantly, some of the earliest welfare reforms concerned workers' compensation for accidents and injury at work, since both workers and their families often became economically dependent on Poor Law provision as a result. Undoubtedly however the restructuring of productive activity away from heavy industries such as coal and steel during the twentieth century has reduced the absolute level of workplace accidents.

Accidents and injuries also occur in other environments. Notable this century have been fatalities and injuries associated with the car, which, because cars are a form of private transport, have been less thoroughly investigated than those associated with the various forms of public transport. In 1996 nearly a quarter of a million people were injured in road accidents, with more than 3,000 deaths (Secretary of State for Health 1998a: 65). Accidents and injuries in the home are also significant, with fire an important hazard which has come under increasing control with changes in the construction of building and sources of energy in the home—electricity and gas are less dangerous than coal fires as forms of heating—as well as smoke alarms. Overall in 1996 there was an accident rate (an accident defined as one requiring some form of medical attention) amongst adults of 21 per 100 men and 15 per 100 women, and amongst children of 31 per 100 boys and 22 per 100 girls, with accident rates typically highest amongst rural populations. The protection of children from accidents whilst allowing them sufficient freedom is particularly difficult.

Type 4 explanations: social relations and subjectivity

The fourth and final type of explanatory approach to health and illness focuses on social relations—on the character of the social life in a given society—and on human subjectivity. The distinction between the material environment on the one hand and social relations is not exact. I have included under the heading of the material environment those features of the world in which people live which, though shaped by human endeavour and consequently by social relations, have a clear material existence and operate on human health directly through the body. Under the heading of social relations and subjectivity I include features of social organization and social relations that relate to social rather than bodily needs, whose impact on health and illness is mediated by mind and subjective experience rather than acting directly on the body (though there can be no human consciousness without bodily processes). It is this mediation via subjectivity that marks the decisive contrast between the two explanations. For example, in the form of resource distribution social inequality can have a direct impact on health via the body, as when poverty exposes an individual to more infectious diseases or means that their diet is in some way inadequate. But poverty can also have an impact on health by lowering self-esteem or increasing feelings of insecurity and in turn affecting an individual's resistance to disease through the immune system. Here there is a psychological mediation absent in the first case. This distinction in the mediating mechanisms is often captured by talking of material and psychological explanations of health; however, since the term 'psychological' tends to suggest a focus on the individual not the societal level, I prefer to contrast the material with the social mediated through consciousness and subjectivity. I have avoided the term 'cultural' because it suggests that it is shared ideas and beliefs that are decisive, whereas I want to ground subjectivity in social relations, structures, and organization, not just cultural values and beliefs. The pathway linking social relations to health and illness is set out in Figure 2.5.

The way in which social relations in a society can exert their impact on health via subjectivity has been a theme of a range of writers. Vicente Navarro (1976), in his Marxist analysis of the impact of capitalism on health, argued that illness was a response both to material conditions and to the subjective alienation associated with wage labour.[11] In so doing he followed Marx in the attention he gave to the productive process. The sort of working conditions that he had in mind were of Fordist factory work, where workers had to carry out a narrow range of repetitive tasks and had little control over their work. They were treated merely as labour power and were in a situation of economic dependence *vis-à-vis* the capitalists who employed them. The conditions under which they worked led to feelings of alienation which Blauner (1964: ch. 2) had earlier characterized in terms of four dimensions—a sense of powerlessness, a lack of meaning and significance in their work, social alienation, and self-estrangement—dimensions which were the inverse of control, purpose, social integration, and self-involvement. Alienation in Navarro's analysis, as in Blauner's, is treated as a subjective experience, and for Navarro it is associated with both physical and mental ill-health. At the individual level this is a Type 2(c) pathway, in which psychological stress mediates directly between the individual's attributes and circumstances and illness, generating a weakened resistance to disease.

Figure 2.5 Type 4 explanations: social relations and subjectivity

Social relations → Subjectivity → Bodily vulnerability → Health/illness

Such ideas, though not necessarily grounded in Marxist formulations, have recently been reaffirmed in a range of studies that emphasize the importance of the degree of control workers have over their jobs and provide evidence that this is linked to their health (Marmot et al. 1997; Bosma et al. 1997)

There is, however, an alternative mechanism. The alienation and stress of wage labour may also lead people to buy and consume products which are themselves unhealthy. For example, Navarro views heavy drinking and heavy smoking as ways in which the individual tries to deal with the stress and unpleasantness of their lives, and in so doing makes ill-health more likely. Here, their behaviour is no longer seen as a free choice by the individual but as a structured, constrained choice that attempts to deal with the difficulties of their individual circumstances, and the shift to the societal level makes the 'risk' behaviour more explicable. This alternative mechanism might be said more properly to belong to Type 3 explanations, since there is a mediation via individual behaviour that acts on the body. However, since stress is so central to the pathogenic processes that are operating and plays a part in generating ill-health by reducing resistance to disease, as well as leading to behaviours that make ill-health more likely, I have treated this type of explanation as belonging to the Type 4 category. In fact what we have in this situation is the interaction of two types of causal mechanism which in combination are likely to make the individual especially vulnerable to ill-health.

The idea that individual behaviours which make ill-health more likely are ways of coping with the stresses of individuals' lives is found in a range of sociological accounts of health and illness. Hilary Graham (1987), for example, argues that women in low-income households with unemployed partners, or as lone mothers, are more likely to smoke because for them smoking is a way of coping with the difficulties of their situations: smoking is a rational action, notwithstanding their lack of resources, since the short-term benefits of helping them to cope with their situation outweigh the additional pressure on their resources and the long-term health risks—smoking is a survival mechanism. A similar argument can be used in relation to the use of psychotropic drugs prescribed by doctors which women may use to cope with the stresses and strains of their lives—sometimes at the price of drug dependence (Ettorre and Riska 1995).

Navarro, like others, also suggests that capitalism itself encourages patterns of consumption like this which play on individuals' psychological vulnerability, since capitalists have an interest in maintaining and enhancing the demand for their products. Consequently alcohol, tobacco, drug, and food companies deploy a range of devices to expand the markets for their products, often emphasizing their associations with leisure and relaxation: a tempting scenario for those facing difficulties in their lives who are looking for ways of relieving stress and anxiety. The marketing of both alcohol and cigarettes as products that are smart and cool and associated with pleasure are obvious instances. So, too, is the focus on slimness and dieting for women, in which having a slender body is held up as the solution to life's potential difficulties for young women—cultural pressures which may make those facing stresses in their life more vulnerable to eating disorders such as anorexia nervosa (Bordo 1990).

Somewhat similar ideas have been developed in a rather different direction by those who characterize the late modern society as the 'risk society', one in which individuals find their lives are increasingly governed by uncertainty and anxiety. Here the focus is primarily on the culture of 'modernity' or 'late modernity', though there is passing reference to industrialism and capitalism as key dimensions of modernity. Giddens, for instance, asserts:

> Modernity is a risk society. I do not mean by this that social life is inherently more risky that it used to be; for most people in developed societies that is not the case. Rather the concept or risk becomes fundamental to the way both lay actors and technical specialists organise the social world. Under the conditions of modernity the future is continually drawn into the present by means of a reflexive organisation of knowledge environments. A territory is carved out and colonised. (1991: 3–1).

Risk assessment, he goes on to argue, 'invites precision, and even quanitification, but by its nature is imperfect'. In this situation of increased uncertainty, anxiety and personal meaninglessness, psychological problems are more common. Anorexia nervosa is the paradigmatic illness of late modern societies, since eating and control of the body become so bound up with self-identity: 'Anorexia represents a striving for security in a world of plural, but ambiguous options' (1991: 107).

In his book *Unhealthy Societies*, Richard Wilkinson (1996) has adopted a rather different approach from that of Navarro or of theorists of the risk society such as Giddens, but one which also focuses on the impact of social relations on health via the mediation of psychological processes. Wilkinson argues that in developed societies, where infectious diseases are no longer the major cause of death, the degree of social cohesion plays a crucial role in explaining levels of health and illness and is mediated by psychological states such as stress.[12] In his view, social cohesion is itself a product of the degree of social inequality in the society, and where inequality is high individuals' feelings of social deprivation, powerlessness, and insecurity are increased with adverse consequences for their health. Where incomes are distributed more equitably, stress is lower and the health of the population is better than where income differences are greater. For Wilkinson, therefore, in advanced industrial societies the force of social inequality as regards ill-health is not that those with low incomes do not have enough material resources for an adequate diet, but that they feel deprived and powerless relative to other people, and that it is these feelings that make them sick. Similarly, the unemployed do not become ill because they cannot feed themselves, but because they feel insecure, their sense of self-worth is diminished, and they become more isolated. The mediation is psycho-social rather than material and bodily, and there is a recognition of individuals' psycho-social as well as bodily needs. The nature of these psycho-social linkages have been discussed further by Williams (1998) in a recent paper in which he argues that the emotions need to be placed centre stage.

Wilkinson's focus on social cohesion and social integration and on feelings of relative deprivation and insecurity, though it is relatively untheorized, has clear echoes of Durkheim's analysis of suicide to which he refers, and introduces an important dimension which exclusive concentration on material conditions acting on the body leaves out. In his first book, *The Division of Labour* (1964 [1893]), Durkheim had explored the foundations of social order and had contended that societies are characterized by one of two types of solidarity. Simpler societies are integrated by what he termed 'mechanical solidarity'. There are few specialized social institutions, and kinship provides the means of organizing social activities. There is a shared consciousness, and individuals are in effect interchangeable units: 'every consciousness beats as one.' In more complex societies, where roles are more highly differentiated as a result of the division of labour, it is the interdependence of people that binds them together like the differing parts of the body. Hence solidarity is organic, and it is the division of labour rather than a common consciousness that holds people together. Moral consciousness still exists, but is less complete and less cohesive. Crime has an important part to play, since it helps to define and clarify the frontiers of what is acceptable but also pushes forward the frontiers of morality. In such societies the regulation of society can be disrupted under conditions of social upheaval such as those generated by economic crises. Under these conditions customs and conventions break down and a state of normlessness, which Durkheim termed 'anomie', can develop. These are the conditions that can lead to what he termed 'anomic suicide', when the rules that set limits on individual's aspirations and desires collapse and the individual in a state of confusion commits suicide. Social integration is important not just for the society as a whole but for the individual.

Wilkinson accepts Durkheim's emphasis on the importance of social integration and on the negative consequences for the individual of a lack of a sense of social cohesion. For Wilkinson, the level of social inequality is crucial to social integration and when social inequality increases social cohesion declines, with adverse psychological consequences for the individual in terms of stress—a stress that itself generates both psychological and physical illness. When income differentials are reduced and cohesion is enhanced, as during the First and Second World Wars in Britain, then the population becomes healthier. Here Wilkinson takes issue with the thesis that it was improvements in diet as a result of rationing that led to improvements in health, noting too that living standards declined during both wars. He contends that it was the reductions in income inequalities and in unemployment along with the sense of cohesion that were decisive.

Wilkinson lists other instances of social groups distinguished by high social cohesion and good health: the community of Italian-Americans in Roseto, eastern Pennsylvania, from the 1930s through to the mid-1960s; certain regions of Italy; and eastern Europe in the 1970s and 1980s. In the next chapter I look in more detail at the way in which he attempts to substantiate his case, arguing that his claim that it is primarily if not exclusively the degree of social inequality and the level of social cohesion that determine levels of health and illness in advanced industrial societies gives too little importance to material factors. However, Wilkinson is right to draw attention to the importance of social cohesion (we can note in this context that rationing may have a dual impact on health by improving diets for some and also serving to strengthen as well as reflect social solidarity). For example, it is striking that, as I noted earlier, the married tend be healthier than the divorced, separated, and widowed. The finding can be analysed at the individual level in terms of marital status, stress, and level of social support. At the societal level, Durkheim's arguments about social cohesion and the problems generated by normlessness provide an analysis that directs us to focus on the family as a social institution, on changing patterns of marital breakdown, and on household composition (the present shift to single-person households is very marked) and on the consequences of all of these for individuals.[13] Durkheim's approach has been criticized because it tended to stress the value for society as a whole of institutions like the family, and the same point could be made about Wilkinson. An interest in social relations and social cohesion should not blind us to the extensive evidence that in advanced industrial societies the nuclear family does not only play a positive role—as a haven in a heartless world (Lasch 1979). It can also often be the source of exploitation and abuse, which can generate physical and psychological ill-health—sexual abuse, for example, is a major cause of psychological disorder. Here the type of Marxist analysis we find in Navarro, as well as feminist analyses of gender division of labour, can be used to counterbalance the Durkheimian picture of the family, since we would expect the alienation of capitalist workers to spill over into the domestic environment.

An important common feature of the accounts of Navarro, Giddens, and Wilkinson is that they specify linkages between the character of society, individuals' psychological experiences, and patterns of health and illness. More often, the way in which the features of society shape individuals' experiences is left out of the analysis. Put another way, the analysis is at the level of the individual, not the society. What is important is the way in which social structures and social relations frame the social circumstances and psychological experiences in people's lives. Cultural factors play a part here, since they help to shape individual consciousness; but analysis at the cultural level needs to be linked to social relations.

Conclusion

The four types of account outlined in this chapter should not be regarded as mutually exclusive alternatives; in particular, analyses at the individual and the societal level complement one another. Yet, whilst complementary, the accounts have very important differences in emphasis. Analyses that focus on individual behaviour stress what the individual can do to affect the pattern of health and illness they experience, whereas those that point to individual attributes and circumstances assume that it is the attributes individuals have and the circumstances in which they find themselves that influence their health status, whether these are matters of genetic inheritance, family transmission (social class and education), or social and political circumstances. In either case, the limitation is that insufficient attention is paid to the way in which material circumstances and social relations at the societal level constrain and shape people's lives, including their health.

Analyses that focus on the material environment of the society and resource distribution place individual behaviour, attributes, and circumstances into a broader context, illuminating how, for instance, the activities of global corporations can influence health. The focus on social relations and subjectivity also brings in the broader societal context, drawing attention to issues such as social cohesion and social integration. In both cases, processes at the individual level, whether of behaviour, attributes, or circumstances, play a mediating role between the societal level forces and health and illness. The precise balance of factors implicated depends on the difference we wish to explain. Whatever the pattern of health and illness under consideration, an important part of the sociologist's contribution is to show the way in which societal forces shape what happens at the individual level. In the next chapter I consider how we can use these different approaches to help us explain the patterns of health and illness outlined in Chapter 1.

Chapter 3

Explaining Trends and Inequalities in Health

IN the previous chapter I distinguished four types of explanatory account of patterns of health and illness. At the individual level they focused either on behaviour or on attributes and circumstances; at the societal level either on the material environment and the body or on social relations and subjectivity. In this chapter I use these accounts to seek to explain some of the particular patterns of health and illness I described in the first chapter. I concentrate on three: long-term improvements in health, class inequalities in health and illness, and gender inequalities.[1]

In looking at these three areas, particularly that of long-term improvements in health, it is necessary to introduce a further factor: the impact of medical interventions on health and illness. So far my examination of types of explanatory account has concentrated on factors that make the occurrence of illness more or less likely. Medical interventions are primarily relevant to patterns of health and illness because they have an impact on the duration and outcome of illness.[2] Inoculation and vaccination are exceptions, since they act to increase resistance to a specific infectious disease and so reduce the likelihood of its occurrence rather than acting on the course of the illness; they can be included either as part of the material environment at the societal level or as a possible individual-level attribute/circumstance.

Long-term trends in health

Drawing on the accounts set out in Chapter 2, it is easy to identify some of the factors which have led to the long-term improvements in the health of the British population that characterize the epidemiological transition which occurred during the 200 years from the mid-eighteenth to the mid-twentieth century. Although separating out the precise balance of factors is not always easy, it is clear that improvements in the material environment resulting from economic changes were crucial. Thomas McKeown, in his highly influential book *The Modern Rise of Population* (1976), argued that the long-term improvements in the health of the British population, visible from the eighteenth century onwards and manifest in reduced mortality from infectious diseases, owed relatively little to developments in medicine or improvements in health services. This, he contended, was demonstrated by the fact that the significant declines in death rates from specific infectious diseases almost always occurred *before* the relevant vaccination, inoculation, or effective drug treatment became available (he provided graphs of the declines in mortality from a range of infectious diseases, noting where the new medical intervention became available to back up this claim). Instead, improvements in 'standards of living' and especially in the nutritional state of the population, which increased the resistance to infections, were crucial, particularly in the eighteenth and first half of the nineteenth century. Nutritional improvements resulted from improvements in food supplies arising from the agricultural revolution and from increases in per capita income. In the second half of the nineteenth century improvements in sanitation, which reduced the spread of water-borne diseases, were also important, and in the twentieth century improvements in personal hygiene and the cleanliness of food also played a part.

McKeown's thesis that developments in medicine did not have much impact on the population's health until well into the twentieth century has been widely accepted. However, the impact of medical advances has been greater in the second half of this century, though even here the highest estimates of their impact suggest that they have added at most five years to average life expectancy over the postwar period (see Wilkinson 1996: 31)—roughly half the gain in life expectancy during this time and only around one-seventh of the gain over the last 150 years. More contentious is McKeown's precise analysis of the other possible factors that generated the long-term decline, with particular controversy over his emphasis on nutrition rather than public hygiene. Certainly there can be no doubt of the correlation that exists between economic growth (measured in terms of the per capita Gross Domestic Product of a country) and improvements in mortality, and in that respect industrialization, including capitalist industrialization, has had long-term benefits for health. However, economic growth measured in terms of GDP is a crude indicator which, for instance, almost certainly underestimates long-term improvements in standards in living (Wilkinson 1996: ch. 3). This is because technological developments which generate improvements in standards of living often become relatively inexpensive after their initial introduction—fridges, important to food hygiene, are a good example. Moreover, a measure of GDP does not tell us about the precise trajectory of particular changes in the material environment which are beneficial to health, nor does it tell us about the distribution of resources within the population. I want, therefore, to look at the key aspects of the material environment identified in the previous chapter—food production, water supply, air pollution—and at resource distribution, putting them in the context of changes in the political and economic organization of society in order to examine their importance in explaining long-term improvements in health.

At the beginning of the eighteenth century landowners were the dominant group in political and economic life in Britain. Landownership was highly concentrated, landlords owning perhaps three-quarters of the cultivated land, and most agriculture was geared to production for the market—there was no longer a real peasantry (Hobsbawm 1969: 98). The population was expanding rapidly and the country was becoming increasingly urbanized imposing further demands on the production and distribution of food (no more than one-third of the employed population worked on the land, and it accounted for only one-third of national income). Yet almost all food consumed in Britain was produced here (transport and conservation made the importation of food difficult); even by the 1830s at least 90 per cent of food consumed in Britain was home-produced. Consequently, the demands on food production were considerable.

During the eighteenth century, however, the supply of food improved and this helped to offset some of the problems associated with urbanization. McKeown (1976: 130–3) lists some of the agricultural advances that underpinned the improvement in food supplies in eighteenth century Britain. These involved an extension of traditional methods of agriculture—increased land use, manuring, winter-feeding, and rotation of crops. This extension was facilitated by a number of changes, including the enclosure movement, changes which together enabled more efficient farming and the exploitation of developments in technology, including crop rotation, the introduction of new crops such as the potato, improved seed production, and developments in transport. However, improved food for the majority went alongside severe difficulties for some. The locally organized Poor Law system provided some redress for those without means of support, but there was a growing surplus of rural poor, some of whom sought work in urban areas, thus fuelling the growth of the towns and cities.

In the nineteenth century food productivity increased yet further. Initially this was through the continuation and extension of traditional methods, but soon new scientific developments associated with industrial revolution began to have an impact, as Hobsbawm describes:

> 'Under-drainage'—essential to bring the heavy and soggy clay-lands into cultivation—spread from the 1820s; in 1843 the cylindrical clay drainpipe was invented. Fertilizers came into use rapidly: superphosphate was patented in 1842, and within the first seven years of the 1840s the import of Peruvian guano rose from virtually zero to over 200,000 tons. 'High farming', with its heavy investment and relative mechanization, dominated the middle years of the century, and from about 1837 the increase in the yield of crops became rather striking. British farming, after seventy years of expansion before 1815 and two or three hesitant decades, entered its golden age. (1969: 106)

The precise consequences of the improvements in agriculture varied across the population. Whilst average nutritional standards were rising, there can be little doubt of the poor diets of large sections of both rural and urban populations in the nineteenth century at a time when an increasing proportion of the population were dependent on wage labour. The staples were bread, potatoes, and tea, the balance between bread and potatoes shifting as the century progressed, when the quantities of potatoes produced increased. Individual consumption of meat was often limited (in 1863, 23 per cent of silk workers in Macclesfield and 17 per cent of the labourers in Coventry had never tasted meat: Wohl 1983: 50). Diets were especially low in protein, lacking in fresh green vegetables and fresh milk and in several vitamins, notably vitamins C and D. The price of food, low wages, endemic underemployment, and the attendant poverty led to under-nourishment across much of the population notwithstanding average improvements.

There were also differences within families as well as across social classes, since food was distributed very unevenly within them. Men, who were most likely to have manual jobs making heavy demands on their bodies and who had higher mortality, tended to consume more of the available food, especially the most nutritious items containing protein such as meat, bacon, eggs, fish, and cheese, since their health was essential to the maintenance of the family wage. This had adverse consequences for women and children. Poorly nourished pregnant women, often suffering from anaemia or rickets, gave birth to low-weight, premature, ill-nourished babies whose own fitness and chances of survival were diminished as a result. The fact that many women also had multiple pregnancies and large families further compounded the situation. In this way poor physical constitution was passed on from one generation to the next not through genetic inheritance but through the inadequacy of nutrition, which usually began for the new generation at the point of conception.

The inadequate diets of many of the population, with their deficiencies in protein and vitamins, were made worse by the fact that much food was adulterated, often through the use of poisonous additives designed to reduce the cost of production or to act as some form of preservative. Here the spread of mass production during the nineteenth century made things worse:

the mass production and marketing techniques developed in the period, the anonymity afforded in the urban setting, and the scale of operations called for by the large, densely packed urban populations, combined to increase the scale and range of adulteration. (Wohl, 1983: 52)

Commercially produced bread, the main staple of the diet of the working class in the country as well as the towns, often contained considerable quantities of alum, which lowered the nutritional value of other foods. Copper was added to some butter to improve its colour, sulphate of iron to tea and beer, and so forth. Wohl comments: 'the list of poisonous additives reads like the stock list of some mad and malevolent chemist' (1983: 53). And if a food was not adulterated by some chemical additive it might be contaminated by infectious micro-organisms due to lack of hygiene in its preparation, transportation or conservation. Milk was particularly liable to adulteration—in 1877 a quarter of all milk was found to be seriously adulterated (Wohl 1983: 21), and in 1862 it was established that over a fifth of all butcher's meat in England and Wales came from diseased animals (p. 53).

It was not until the final quarter of the nineteenth century, and particularly the final decade, that the diets of the working class population improved significantly, and initially this had particular benefits for the health of those aged 15–45 (Blane 1987). During this period, though wages were falling, the price of the staple foods actually declined by 30 per cent, and by the end of the century consumption of sugar, meat, and milk had increased.[3] Much of this decline in price resulted from a rapid expansion in food imports during the final decades of the nineteenth century. The opening up of the American railway system, completed in 1866, facilitated the importation of American wheat into what was by then a free-trade Britain, halving its price between the years 1873 and 1893. Canned meat also began to be imported from America during the same period, though its cheapness was matched by poor quality; however, from the 1880s the introduction of refrigerated steamships increased the imports in meat from the US, the Argentine and New Zealand very rapidly and led to a revolution in the diet of the working classes (Burnett 1968: 134). Yet even by the end of the century estimates suggest some 40 per cent of the working class (by far the largest group in the population) were malnourished (Blane 1987).

In addition, there were greater efforts to reduce the adulteration of food, though fines for those found guilty were often small. The first Adulteration of Foods Act of 1860 was ineffective, but after various amendments it was replaced by the Sale of Food and Drugs Act of 1875 which, though much amended, still provides the basis of the current law (Burnett 1968: 257–60). Significant, too, was a new recognition that the marketing of food free from adulteration could be turned to producers' and sellers' commercial advantage, and companies began to emphasize the purity of their products, a cultural and commercial shift that did much to reduce adulteration.

Against this general background of overall improvements in agriculture and some reduction in the adulteration of food in the second half of the nineteenth century, which were sufficient to benefit the overall health of the population but affected the working class population only slowly, have to be set the adverse effects of the industrial revolution on working conditions and the environment. Whilst the industrial revolution was associated with rapid economic growth (indeed partly defined by it), it initially had a number of other direct, adverse effects for health, particularly the health of the labouring populations in towns and cities. Much of this was linked to the development of new forms of industrial processes in factories or with the expansion of other industries such as coal mining. Early industrialization was associated with severe exploitation of the labour force in which their health and safety were of little concern. There was an over-supply of labour, much work was unskilled, and a sick or injured worker could readily be replaced by another. Long hours meant that fatigue was a major problem, workers were exposed to dangerous substances, and ventilation was often exceptionally poor. In the later 1840s and early part of the 1850s life expectancy actually declined a little (see Table 1.1).

Various substances that had very severe consequences for health were in common use in manufacturing in the nineteenth century. These included substances containing arsenic, white phosphorus, which was used widely in making matches, lead, which was widely used in printing, painting, and the manufacture of earthenware and floor coverings such as linoleum, and chlorine, used in bleaching. Depending on the industrial process in question, workers commonly developed their own distinctive types of ill-health and disablement—occupational diseases—that reflected their type of work. Anthony Wohl, in his vivid portrayal of public health in the second half of the nineteenth century, *Endangered Lives*, describes some of them:

> Miner's asthma, or, as it was more graphically called, 'black spit', potter's asthma, or 'potter's rot', brass-founder's ague, or 'Monday fever', matchmaker's necrosis, or 'phossy jaw', cutlery grinder's asthma and chimney sweep's cancer, or 'soot wart'—these and many more were all part and parcel of the Victorian vocabulary. One did not have to have the penetrating acumen of a Sherlock Holmes to detect the specific trades of various working men. The tailor was betrayed by his concave chest and stooped shoulders, the file-maker by his paralyzed wrist or thumb, the matchmaker by his (or her) teeth or jaw, the miner by his calloused knees and elbows and bad eyes, the potter by his asthma, the lead worker by his paralyzed wrist, the brass worker and copper worker by the tell-tale greenish tint of the hair, teeth, and clothing, the pottery and earthenware worker by his blue gums, the worker handling mercury by his 'trembles', and the confectionery worker by the skin boils which were the first sign of arsenical poisoning (1983: 264–5).

Data on deaths from respiratory disease by occupation provide some evidence of the impact of working conditions on workers' health, although differences in the age structure of the groups and their physical fitness arising from nutritional standards will also have contributed to the mortality differences (coal miners' mortality rates were comparatively low because young, fit men tended to go down the mines and they were better nourished because of higher wages). Table 3.1 gives data provided by the Registrar-General as late as 1897 and shows the marked occupational differences in death levels from respiratory disease.

Women, of course—even if they did not work in these industries, and many textile workers were women—did not entirely escape the direct impact of dangerous substances, which were brought into their houses on the bodies and clothes of their husbands, brothers, or fathers.[4] And the same applied to children.

In addition to the ill-health and premature mortality generated by working with dangerous substances, workers also faced the danger of injury or even death in their working environments as a result of 'accidents'. Workers in the textile industry were quite frequently maimed or incapacitated by machinery,

Table 3.1 Deaths from diseases of the respiratory system by occupation, 1897

Occupation	Deaths
Agricultural workers	100
Coal Miners	133
Wool manufacturers	202
Cotton manufacturers	244
Lead workers	247
Chimney sweeps	249
Brass workers	250
Zinc workers	266
Copper miners	307
Copper workers	317
Lead miners	319
File makers	373
Tin miners	400
Cutlery, scissor-makers	407
Potters, earthenware workers	453

Data are for male workers, and use a base figure of 100 for agricultural workers for comparative purposes.

Source: Registrar General 1897, in Wohl (1983: 282).

and some were killed. The same was true of miners. Copper, lead, and tin miners all had high death rates, and although coal miners had death rates below those of the average working man because they were such a highly selected group (young, strong, and healthy as well as relatively well paid), nonetheless their deaths from accidents were still high.

In the nineteenth century the regulation of manufacturing was limited, and the major health hazards facing workers were not controlled at all successfully. There were various attempts to regulate factory conditions, including the length of the working day and levels of ventilation, but most of the measures had little impact. White phosphorus, though banned in several other European countries, was not banned in Britain till 1910, and it was only in 1895 that a Factory and Workshop Act required the notification of industrial diseases and a Home Office Dangerous Substances Committee was established to examine actual or potentially harmful industrial processes (Wohl 1983: 267). A Workmen's Compensation Act was passed in 1897 which was designed to improve safety and reduce accidents by putting their cost at the employers' door. However, there is little evidence of a direct, positive effect on safety (see Bartrip 1985).

One change of particular significance was the growing exclusion of women (especially married women) and children from the paid labour market. From the 1840s women began to be excluded by legislation from the most dangerous forms of paid work, and during the second half of the century middle-class notions of respectability helped to keep many married women outside the paid labour force (though unfortunately nineteenth-century data on female participation in the labour market are not very good (Lewis 1983)). This exclusion resulted from a number of factors including the threat posed by women workers to male wages (married women in particular were willing to work for lower wages). In itself the loss of women's wages would have reduced family income and lowered nutritional standards. However, it was associated with demands by men for a 'family wage'—a male wage sufficient to cover the whole family which helped to compensate for the loss of women's income (Barrett and McIntosh 1980), so that overall working-class women's health may have benefited from the exclusion.

One area where clear progress was made in the second half of the nineteenth century was in the cleanliness of water and sanitation. Rapid urbanization and industrialization posed enormous problems for the supply of clean water and personal hygiene because of the density of populations and the problems generated for the disposal of human excrement. Wohl comments: 'Among the many problems which urban densities exacerbated none was greater than the accumulation of human excrement, both human and animal' (1983: 80).

In rural areas sanitary provision was also generally poor and posed problems for human hygiene; the majority of water came from local wells, excrement was dumped into cesspools and there was often little separation of animals from humans. Writing in 1864 John Simon summarized the findings of the Privy Council on rural sanitation:

> The most various accumulations of animal filth in close proximity to dwellings, entire absence of drainage, and drains inoperative and stinking, ponds and ditches equivalent to open cesspools, drinking-water polluted and made poisonous with refuse—such are the evils which .... local authorities are doing nothing, or nothing adequate, to remove. (quoted in Wohl, 1983: 92)

In towns and cities the problems were multiplied and population density led to contamination. Initially, as towns and cities grew most of the excrement was dumped in the street or in stone cesspools which were rarely cleaned, so adjoining land became saturated and wells contaminated. Unpleasant smells were a feature of urban life.

The lack of water to domestic dwellings (in the 1840s only about 20 per cent of houses in Birmingham had piped water and only 10 per cent in Newcastle; in 1879 over one-quarter of all local authorities had no piped water whatever) meant that even without the problem of sewage, for many people cleanliness was difficult to achieve, even though most put considerable effort into it (the sale of soaps and disinfectants increased considerably in the second half on the nineteenth century, but again the poor were disadvantaged because of the cost).

However, by the second half of the nineteenth century public health interventions began to have some impact. Of particular importance were gradual improvements in the disposal of excrement. These tended to take place in three stages. In the first place, cesspools were drained, cleaned and made watertight; in the second stage a system of dry conservancy was introduced into homes to deal with human excrement; and thirdly, once piped water had been introduced, water closets were used to dispose of excrement. In addition, municipal baths, often ornate in design and construction, began to be built from the 1840s onwards; they were an important symbol of municipal endeavour, and were quite widely used (significantly more by men than women, and more were provided for men, a difference attributable both to men's greater involvement in dirty work as well as cost).

Important though they were, improvements in sanitation would have had even more impact were it not for the poor nourishment of a significant proportion of the population despite average improvements. Nonetheless, by the end of the nineteenth century there were clear signs of overall improvements in health measured in terms of longevity, and life expectancy had increased about eight years on average since the early 1840s, though there was little change in infant mortality until the twentieth century and in mortality amongst the over 45s until the 1890s.

Improvements in mortality in Britain in the first half of the twentieth century, when the largest gains in life expectancy took place, were brought about by further changes in many of the same factors. In the first place, the living standards of the working-class population continued to improve in relation both to nutritional standards and to sanitation. A number of factors underpinned these improvements. First, despite the fact that the period was characterized by a loss of dynamism in the British economy and economic depression during the 1920s and 1930s, which increased levels of unemployment (employment had increased significantly between 1890 and 1914) and kept wage levels down, the cost of living declined. By 1914 over half of Britain's food supplies were imported and prices of imported foods fell considerably so that the total cost of food was reduced.[5] An average working-class family spent 60 per cent of its income on food in 1914; by 1938–9 this figure had fallen to 35 per cent (Constantine 1977: 24).

The First World War led to concerns about Britain's heavy dependence on food imports and calls for an increase in domestic production. In the event, however, the rise in standards of living in the interwar period led to increased demand not for staples like bread and potatoes but for more expensive foods rich in nutrients like high-quality meat, eggs, fruit, and green vegetables, which British farmers were in a better position to supply (it was hard for them to compete in supplying grain at competitive prices). The effect of these changes on the average diet was significant, even though there were many who could not afford the more expensive foodstuffs.

In addition, there was greater regulation of the food industry as well as improvements in conservation so that adulteration and contamination of food became less common. Whilst pasteurization of milk was not introduced until after the Second World War, there were other developments that helped to reduce contamination. Refrigeration had been introduced in the 1880s and began to be important in the transportation of food (it was one factor that helped to increase the quantity of imported food), though it was not common in private homes until the 1950s, when the acquisition of a domestic fridge became part of the new postwar affluence (with around 30 per cent of households then owning one (Hobsbawm 1969: 263).

Another factor raising average standards of living and reducing the cost of food to families was the marked decline in family size, which had begun in the middle classes in the 1870s but included the working classes during the first half of the twentieth century. Table 3.2 shows the striking decline in completed family size of women marrying in the late 1930s when compared with those marrying in the 1860s.

This reduction in average family size not only contributed to the overall health of the family by reducing the demands on wages, so allowing nutritional

Table 3.2 Completed family size, England and Wales, marriage cohorts 1861–1939

Marriage cohort	Family size	Marriage cohort	Family size
1861–9	6.16	1910–14	2.82
1871	5.94	1915–19	2.46
1876	5.62	1920–4	2.31
1881	5.27	1925–9	2.11
1896	4.81	1930–4	2.07
1900–9	3.30	1935–9	2.03

Mean ultimate family size of marriages contracted when the woman was under 45.

Source: Busfield and Paddon (1977)

standards to rise, it also had profound consequences for the health of women who were especially susceptible to death and illness if they continued to have frequent pregnancies.[6] Of women marrying in 1870–9 over 50 per cent had six or more children; of women marrying in 1925 only 7 per cent did so. Moreover, with the exception of wartime, during the first half of this century only around 10 per cent of married women were in paid work, a factor that may have had some benefits for their health given typical working conditions, though it put pressure on resources in poor families.[7]

A further factor contributing to the improvement in standards of living in the first half of the twentieth century were a range of Liberal welfare reforms over the period 1906–14. These reforms centred on the National Insurance Act of 1911, which introduced mandatory unemployment and sickness state insurance schemes to provide some financial cover as well as primary medical care for men working in specific industries—a list that was rapidly extended—with contributions from employees, employers, and the state.[8] Also important was the 1908 Pensions Act, which introduced non-contributory pensions for those aged 70 and over with a reduction for any wages being earned—a measure helpful to the standards of living of the elderly whose survival depended on their current as well as past social circumstances.

The Liberal legislation of this period also included a set of measures related to children's health which was increasingly seen as the responsibility of mothers at home who, it was argued, needed to be educated in matters of child welfare. The legislation was prompted by concerns about children's health initially resulting from the detection of very poor standards of physical health amongst potential recruits to the Boer War, about 40 per cent of whom had to be rejected because they did not meet the minimum standards even though the standards were not very high. This led to the establishment of an Interdepartmental Committee on Physical Deterioration whose 1904 report focused particularly on the welfare of infants and children—the next generation—and recommended the provision of school meals and school medical inspections. The 1906 Education (Provision of Meals) Act that followed required local authorities to provide free school meals for children who needed them, and school medical inspections to detect health problems were included in the provisions of an Education Act of 1907. In 1908 a Children's Act was passed which covered a range of issues including juvenile justice and contained a provision making it an offence to sell cigarettes to anyone under the age of 16 (Lewis 1980).

The First World War regenerated the same concerns about the health of children and young adults when it was found that a similar proportion of potential recruits as in the Boer war were graded unfit for service (though the standards applied had been reduced).[9] The Local Government Board issued an order under which mothers and infants were to be provided with free milk by local authorities, the Board paying 50 per cent of the cost. The order was revoked in 1921 when the war had ended, although the next year new regulations were introduced requiring local authorities to provide milk but on a means-tested basis. However, in 1934 a surplus of milk production led the Government to provide cheap milk to school children. In addition, from 1915 Government grants were made to support infant welfare centres operated by local authorities, which provided health inspection for infants and education in child-care for mothers. The 1918 Maternal and Child Welfare Act required local authorities to establish committees to oversee work in this area, and encouraged them to develop maternal and infant welfare services including salaried midwives, health visitors, and infant welfare centres (Lewis 1980: 34).[10] With the Second World War, and a renewed recognition of the importance of the health of mothers and infants, a new national milk scheme was introduced which provided pregnant and nursing mothers and every child under 5 with a free pint of milk as well as vitamin supplements—cod liver oil, rosehip syrup, fruit juice, and pills.

Higher standards of living in the first half of the twentieth century also meant improved housing, including improved water supplies, and sanitation. The question of housing attracted considerable attention during the First World War, and the slogan 'Homes Fit for Heroes' reflected the public support for the building of new houses (there had been a shortage before the war and house-building came to a standstill during the war). Between the two wars some four million new houses were built, over one million by local authorities (Hopkins 1979: 238) (public subsidies also supported some private house-building)—

houses that had more adequate sanitation than the majority of the slums which remained.

Whilst job insecurity and unemployment created very severe problems for some groups during the depression of the 1930s, the overall period also witnessed considerable improvements in working conditions, including hours of work. Important here was the shift away from the traditional manufacturing areas—coal, textiles, and to a lesser extent shipbuilding—where Britain lost its global dominance, to new areas such as engineering and electrical goods, chemicals, and cars and other vehicles, which tended to concentrate on the home market and were not very capable of effective international competition (Hobsbawm 1969: ch. 13). Yet in all these areas output increased dramatically. In addition the commercial and financial sector maintained its strength. Overall this restructuring of manufacturing industry and the growing importance of the financial and commercial sectors meant that fewer people were engaged in the unhealthiest of work environments, a change strengthened by further legislation concerning health and safety at work. Hours of work declined rapidly in the period following the First World War, from the 53–4 hours of the pre-war period to an average 48 hours by 1921 (Hopkins 1979: 228).

Viewed overall, there can be little doubt therefore that the long-term decline in mortality from the mid-eighteenth century to the mid-twentieth century was primarily due to societal-level changes in economic organization and the material environment, changes which had their impact on the circumstances of individuals. The individual health-related behaviours which are often the focus of present-day analyses have little relevance in understanding this epidemiological transition, though they will have accounted for some of the differences in health and illness between individuals. Nor is it likely that issues of social cohesion and subjectivity had much to do with the long-term improvements in health, though again they may have been important in producing health inequalities at a particular point of time. The precise weight of the different components of the material environment is difficult to establish and undoubtedly varied over time; the debates over their relative significance in accounting for long-term changes will certainly continue.

Class inequalities in health

The situation in relation to present-day class inequalities in health is rather different. I noted in the previous chapter that these differences cannot be adequately accounted for in terms of social drift, a process in which those with poorer health end up in lower social positions because of their ill-health. Moreover, the argument for the importance of social factors and subjectivity rather than material factors causing ill-health is rather stronger than it is with long-term trends. The key recent proponent of this type of argument is Richard Wilkinson, who in his *Unhealthy Societies* argues (as I outlined in Chapter 2) that current class inequalities in health in Britain are primarily due to social rather than material factors: in particular it is the feelings of relative deprivation generated by income inequalities and the insecurity of unemployment that are decisive. As he puts it, in societies that have gone through the epidemiological transition, 'What affects health is no longer the differences in absolute material standards but social position within societies' (1996: 75). What matters is not whether you have a larger or smaller house or a car, 'but what these and similar difference means socially and what they make you feel about yourself and the world around you'. The causal pathway is not one of material factors at the societal level acting on the body, perhaps mediated by individual behaviour, but one of societal-level social relations and arrangements which at the individual level are mediated by psychological not bodily processes. However, before turning to examine the empirical support for the alternative societal-level accounts, the role of individual behaviour in accounting for class inequalities in health needs to be considered, since it is often suggested that individual behaviours can account for class differences in health.

There is some evidence of differences in risk behaviour by social class. These are most marked in relation to smoking. Table 3.3 shows the differences in smoking by socio-economic group for men and women. As these data show, men and women in the unskilled manual group are more than twice as likely to

Table 3.3 Prevalence of smoking by socio-economic group, Great Britain, 1994

Socio-economic group	Men	Women
Professional	16	12
Employers and managers	20	20
Intermediate and junior non-manual	24	23
Skilled manual and own account non-professional	33	29
Semi-skilled manual	38	32
Unskilled manual	40	34
All	28	26

% of men and women aged 16 and over.

Source: Bunting (1997: table 15.13)

smoke as those in the professional group, a difference that has increased over the last twenty years.

There is also a class-related pattern of obesity for women but not for men. The data are given in Table 3.4. However, data on physical activity show no very clear overall associations with social class. Whereas the proportion of men and women with activity levels of 'none' increases with social class, high levels of physical activity are more common amongst men from the manual than the non-manual groups, and this is true, though to a lesser extent, amongst women. This class difference in high levels of physical activity is related to the higher levels of work-related activity in the manual groups. The evidence indicates that non-manual groups engage in more physical activity outside the workplace: levels of walking and sports activity are higher in the non-manual than the manual groups amongst both men and women (Bunting 1997: 220)—an observation that fits the data on the class association with those reporting no occasions of even moderate activity.

Data on alcohol consumption provide little evidence that would allow us to account for class differences in mortality in terms of higher alcohol consumption amongst those in the lower social classes: rather the reverse. There is a class gradient for alcohol consumption but for both men and women there is a positive association with higher consumption, with unskilled and semi-skilled workers having the lowest levels of consumption, differences that are more marked for women than men (Bunting 1997: 216).

Taken together, these data show that one or two individual behaviours, most obviously smoking, may contribute to the observed class differences in mortal-

Table 3.4 Prevalence of obesity by social class, England, 1994

Social class	BMI over 25		BMI over 30	
	Men	Women	Men	Women
I	55.3	43.3	9.6	11.7
II	57.5	44.7	12.9	13.0
IIIN	58.2	45.2	13.6	14.5
IIIM	58.9	50.1	14.1	19.1
IV	52.4	53.1	14.6	21.9
V	53.2	54.9	13.2	21.8
All	56.8	48.0	13.3	21.1

Source: Bunting (1997: table 15.15)

Body-mass index of men and women aged 16 and over.

ity. However, they are not sufficient in themselves to account for them—a conclusion supported by data from other studies. The Whitehall study mentioned in the previous chapter indicated that an inverse relation between health and civil service grade remained even when behavioural and other risk factors were taken into account (Marmot et al. 1978). I also noted the qualification about the importance of individual behaviour made as a result of the 1984–5 Health and Lifestyles Survey (Blaxter 1990), which found that if you consider two health related factors—smoking and drinking—abstention makes no difference to those in disadvantageous social circumstances. Put another way it is only amongst those whose circumstances are good where 'healthy' behaviour makes a difference (Blaxter 1990: 216). Bunting concludes her review of morbidity and health-related behaviours with the comment that 'the differences in health-related behaviours by socio-economic status do not explain most of the observed differences in health' (1997: 221).

If class-related differences in individual behaviour can only be part of the explanation of class inequalities in health, what role do social relations play? Is Wilkinson right in claiming that social relations, not material circumstances, are decisive? Certainly he is right in his belief that we should take account of factors such as social cohesion and feelings of deprivation and insecurity, and of their links to social inequality. As I noted in the previous chapter, a range of evidence shows the adverse consequences of psychological stress on health, and stress has been strongly linked to social relations, not only to social support, but also to employment relations and conditions of work (Marmot et al. 1997; Bosma et al. 1997). Wilkinson does not, however, establish satisfactorily that in advanced industrial societies material circumstances no longer make a significant contribution: both material resources and social relations contribute to existing health inequalities. To demonstrate this it is helpful to look first at the way in which Wilkinson tries to substantiate his argument.

Wilkinson's strategy is threefold. First, he analyses data on economic growth, social inequality, and health. Here, he argues that though economic growth is associated with long-term increases in longevity, once societies reach a particular level of income gains in longevity reach a plateau. He also contends that societies with greater social inequality as measured by income inequality have higher levels of mortality than might be expected on the basis of per capita income alone; conversely, countries like Japan, where social inequality is less, have lower levels of mortality. Wilkinson backs up his claim using data on income inequality and health across a range of societies. However, others have argued that whilst there is some association between the extent of income inequality and health, the association is not as strong as Wilkinson claims (Judge et al. 1998). The key issue here relates not to health differences between societies but to health inequalities within the society and to Wilkinson's claim that these are determined by social relations mediated by subjectivity. Yet aggregate-level data do not settle any dispute about the salience of material factors mediated directly by the body versus the salience of social relations mediated by subjectivity in producing the observed health inequalities, since reductions in income inequality will be associated with improvements in the material environment for those towards the bottom of the social structure. Against this Wilkinson contends, using comparative data from Britain and Sweden, that the health of the whole population benefits from reductions in income inequality, not just the poorer groups (in Sweden there is no very clear class gradient in mortality, and mortality is lower than in Britain even in highest-status groups), though the poorest benefit the most. However, these differences could be taken to suggest that both material resources and social relations are important, and the data can hardly be considered decisive since Wilkinson fails to consider possible material reasons for the lower mortality levels of the overall population in Sweden such as better nutritional standards, less atmospheric pollution, better working environments, or less smoking.[11]

Second, in order to support his case Wilkinson examines a number of different societies at specific historical moments where social cohesion has been greater and has, he contends, had a positive impact on health. One of these is Britain during the two world wars. However, Wilkinson wants us to accept that the key factor underpinning the reductions in health inequalities between classes in these two periods was social cohesion generated by reductions in income inequality. Yet here again he does not establish that material factors were of little significance. Although it is striking that sharp declines in mortality and reductions in class inequalities in mortality occurred during both wars, we should not assume that the same factors underpinned the mortality gains on each occasion. I have already noted some of the material factors underpinning the increases in longevity which affected all classes in the first half of the twentieth century, and the fact that the gains were particularly striking during the the First World War no doubt relates at least in part to the rapid social changes associated with the war. This was a period of especially marked declines in family size which enhanced the standards of living of the whole family, of improvements in welfare provisions, as well as very low unemployment (2.8 per cent in July 1914 and only 0.5 per cent in August 1918), and of a two-thirds fall in the numbers reliant on the Poor Law. In the Second World War the declines in unemployment and poverty were also important, as was rationing (as Wilkinson recognizes in an earlier chapter (1996: 54)).[12] He also fails to note that owing to the character of the war itself and popular support for it, social cohesion was almost certainly greater in the Second than the First World War—the epithet 'the people's war' was used both at the time and subsequently to describe the Second World War (Calder 1969). It is true that housing deteriorated, as did medical services, because of the shift of resources away from the civilian population. However, it is arguably sanitation more than housing *per se* that is important to health, and the effect of deteriorating medical services was probably to delay the possible gains from technological developments in medicine rather than to have a direct adverse effect on mortality.[13] Again, therefore, the case that it is greater social cohesion acting on health primarily via psychosocial rather than material pathways that is decisive is not established.

Finally, Wilkinson turns to the data showing associations between feelings of stress and insecurity and poorer health to support his case. Although he is right in seeing such associations as well established (see Chapter 2 above), nonetheless, positive evidence of such associations does not establish that material factors are not important. What we have is a convincing case that issues of social cohesion must be brought into the picture because of the feelings of deprivation and insecurity they generate. We do not have a convincing case that differences in material conditions are not contributing directly to the inequalities.

It is possible to provide a range of evidence indicating the continuing importance of material factors in contributing to class inequalities in health in present-day British society. In order to do so I want to consider the related issues of poverty and unemployment and their consequences for health, as well as the impact of environmental hazards. We can explore the issue of poverty by considering two groups of growing numerical importance both absolutely and relatively. First, lone parents. The proportion of lone parents in Britain has increased significantly over recent years (from 8 per cent of those with dependent children in 1971 to 22 per cent in 1996 (ONS 1998b: table 2.4)), as a result both of the increase of births outside marriage (though growing numbers of couples cohabit) and of the increase in divorce. The majority (over 90 per cent) of lone parents are women, since they are more likely than men to have custody of children and are less likely to remarry. A very high proportion are on benefit—often taken as an indicator of poverty (in 1995–6 some 63 per cent were in receipt of income support (DSS 1997)). Whilst benefit levels are supposed to be sufficient to meet basic material needs, in practice this is only possible if no money is spent on vital social needs. Not surprisingly, studies indicate that lone mothers often have poor diets. And any nutritional deficiencies have an adverse impact not only on their own health but also on that of their children, affecting birth weight and height and subsequent development. This also applies to smoking, which affects their own and their children's health not only through foetal development but also via passive smoking. Predictably, a recent review of the health of lone mothers in Britain found they had worse health than couple mothers and argued that poverty played a crucial role (Shouls et al. 1999).

Second, there are the elderly, the majority of whom are also women.[14] The numbers of those aged 65 and over have also been increasing relatively and absolutely as mortality rates decline and birth rates continue at relatively low levels. They are often excluded from the main calculations on class differences in mortality, yet, as I noted in Chapter 1, class differences in mortality and morbidity in this age group are still striking. Whilst death rates amongst the elderly are partly a function of their earlier experiences, they are also influenced by what happens to them once they have ended their working lives. During old age not only is adequate nutrition essential but so too, as in infancy, is sufficient warmth (as the cases of those dying from hypothermia during the winter months attest). Yet there is clear evidence that poverty is relatively common amongst the elderly, and that this affects diets and levels of heating (Arber and Ginn 1991). One study showed a correlation between pension rates and mortality rates for the elderly and provided some evidence of a causal connection (Wilkinson 1986b).

A further overlapping issue is that of unemployment, though the unemployed, like the elderly, are often excluded from the data showing class differences in mortality and morbidity. Here the evidence is far from conclusive. There can be little doubt that, as we observed in Chapter 2, unemployment increases psychological stress and is associated in particular with higher levels of depression (Warr 1987). Studies of factory closures also show that morbidity is increased in the period of anticipation before redundancy takes effect (Cobb and Kasl 1977). But once individuals become unemployed the evidence as to whether they have higher levels of ill-health and mortality is much more equivocal (Bartley 1993). The unemployed as a group undoubtedly include more people with poorer health, since ill-health is a factor that makes unemployment more likely, but long-term unemployment of two to three years does not appear to increase morbidity levels overall (countervailing tendencies operate: for instance, less exposure to work-related accidents, alongside some increase in stress-related illnesses). However, over an even longer term (around ten years) there is evidence from longitudinal studies of increased mortality. In order to make sense of these apparently contradictory findings Bartley argues that we need to take account of the interaction between the personal characteristics of the individual, including their health, and the state of the labour market (locally as well as nationally), which affects the extent to which those who are less fit and healthy are incorporated into or excluded from employment. She also notes that where jobs are of short duration, as is often the case with unskilled work, the selection of the fittest and healthiest will be enhanced with repetition of the sorting process. If we exclude from the analysis those with severe health problems when they become unemployed, who initially have higher rates of mortality, the mortality rates of the long-term unemployed rise over time because they are in a situation where it is hard for them to meet their biological and social needs adequately—and like lone parents they suffer socially and materially. Stress, Bartley argues, is not the decisive factor.

Finally, we need to consider the continuing effect of differential working environments. Some jobs in manufacturing and in building and construction continue to be more dirty and dangerous than other jobs. Whilst deaths from accidents at work are far lower than they used to be, they have not by any means been eliminated. Moreover, atmospheric and water pollution is concentrated in some localities. A recent study by Blane and his colleagues (1998) looked at the class distribution of six environmental hazards: atmospheric pollution, residential damp, occupational fumes and dusts, physically arduous work, cigarette smoking, and inadequate nutrition, all measured at the individual level, although all linked to the material environment. Although the samples used were small, the authors found that there were class differences in mean scores for both men and women in the expected direction, and the differences remained, though they were marginally smaller, when smoking was removed. The study did not involve any direct attempt to measure health, but the authors note that the difference in exposure to environmental hazards mirrored the social class differences in life expectancy.

There seems little doubt, therefore, that on the basis of a range of evidence it is safe to conclude that material factors make a significant contribution to class differences in mortality and morbidity in Britain. However, unlike the long-term trends, the explanatory importance of social relations and subjectivity does also need to be considered.

Gender inequalities in health

The data presented in Chapter 1 show that gender inequalities in health as measured by longevity are, if anything, even greater than class inequalities. Since mortality and morbidity do not fall neatly into line as they do with the cross-sectional data on age, class, and ethnicity, the picture is more complex and confusing. Any explanation needs to take account of the distinctive combination of women's greater longevity than men's, but reported sickness that is as high or even higher.

The first issue we need to consider is the role of genetically-based biological differences between men and women. The case for the importance of genetic factors in accounting for differences in longevity between the sexes is based primarily on two sets of observations. First, whilst at conception more male foetuses are produced than female (a ratio of some 106 to 100), the chances of survival of male foetuses during pregnancy and the first year of life tend to be lower (in 1996 UK infant mortality was 6.8 per 1,000 births for boys but only 5.4 for girls (ONS 1998a: table 2.20)). Second, in most societies women tend to live longer than men. Taken together, these facts are often used to argue the case for male biological vulnerability and female biological superiority (with the suggestion that the latter is necessary because of the importance of women in reproduction). It is sometimes also argued that, as childbirth has become safer and the number of pregnancies women have to face has declined, women's biological superiority has become more manifest (Hart 1989).

The problem with such arguments, however, is that they tend to treat genetic factors as primary (as *the* explanation) and environmental factors as secondary, as if once we have identified the contribution of genetic factors that is the major part of the explanatory story about gender differences in health, which it clearly is not. The survival of male foetuses depends on an interaction between genes and the environment in the womb and subsequently. For instance, where male offspring are particularly highly valued the survival of female foetuses at birth and during the first year of life is reduced. Moreover, the fact that women are now more likely to survive their childbearing years is due to social rather than genetic factors. We cannot get very far in explaining observed gender inequalities in health without paying adequate attention to social and environmental factors because the gender inequalities in health and longevity are themselves so variable. There are of course biological differences between men and women, and we must in particular pay attention to the impact of reproduction; but above all it is what happens in men's and women's lives that is crucial. For example, it is well established that because of biological differences in body mass and metabolism women should drink less alcohol than men if their performance is not to be impaired. This means that different levels of acceptable alcohol consumption are now set for men and women. Genetically based biological differences are clearly important, but insofar as alcohol consumption affects health it is the social fact of differences in patterns of consumption that is crucial. To what extent, therefore, can gender differences in longevity be accounted for by gender differences in health-related behaviours?

Gender differences in health-related behaviours undoubtedly play some part in gender differences in longevity. In Britain at present men score less well than women on almost all the health-related behaviours included in the current lists. As Table 3.3 above shows, amongst those aged 16 and over in 1994 more men than women were current smokers (28 per cent of men against 26 per cent of women). Men also tend to be heavier smokers (on average 114 cigarettes a week against women's 97) (Bunting 1997: 215). These differences may not seem very large, but they have been declining over time, and current patterns of health will be as much a product of smoking patterns in previous years, when they were somewhat larger, as of the patterns shown in the most recent figures (in 1980 42 per cent of men and 37 per cent of women were current smokers: Townsend and Davidson (1988: 111)).

Men are also more likely to drink heavily than women, even taking into account the different standards set for acceptable alcohol levels for men and women because of biological differences. In 1994 the average weekly consumption of men aged 16 and over was 15.4 units and that for women only 5.4 units (ONS 1997b: table 15.14). Overall, women also have healthier diets than men. The Health and Lifestyle Survey showed marked gender differences in those with 'bad' dietary habits with women having more 'good' dietary habits; however, the same study showed more of them are overweight, again across all classes (Blaxter 1990: 126, 128). However, the latter finding is not supported by data from the 1994 Health Survey for England given in Table 3.4 above, which showed 57 per cent of men aged 16 and over overweight (body mass index over 25) compared with 48 per cent of women, though there were more obese women (BMI over 30)—21 per cent—than obese men—13 per cent. This difference in levels of obesity could be because women tend to have more sedentary lives—one of the health-related behaviours where they score less well than men. The proportion of men with high physical activity levels is greater than that of women largely because of men's higher work-related activity levels (ONS 1999: 128). Men are also more likely to have unprotected sex than women. These differences in health-related behaviour need to be explained; however, they are not sufficient in themselves to account for the gender differences in longevity. Nor do they account for the gender difference in reported sickness.

Central to any understanding of gender differences in longevity and reported morbidity has to be recognition of the gender division of labour both in the workplace and in the family. First, there is the impact on mortality rates of differences in male and female participation in the labour market and the high degree of gender segregation within it. Although the participation of women, especially married women, in the paid labour market has increased very significantly over the last three decades, far more women than men have part-time jobs and spend some period of time out of the labour market having children. Moreover, women tend to have very different jobs from men and tend to be excluded from the most polluting and dangerous jobs such as agricultural labour, mining, and construction, where death rates are higher. For example, in the study of environmental hazards mentioned earlier (Blane et al. 1998) —by no means all related to work—women had lower scores than men for exposure to hazards and the differences were statistically significant. A higher percentage of women in the labour market than men have some form of whitecollar work; they are concentrated in clerical, personal services, sales, and shop work, where typically there are fewer mortality risks from pollution or injury. There is also evidence that men find their paid jobs more alienating than do women, not least because their expectations about their work differ. Insofar as men are more likely to see paid jobs as their key role in life and have higher aspirations, they tend to find work more stressful than women, who are more likely to be motivated by a desire for sociability and social interaction (Martin and Roberts 1984). However, in Britain at present women's wages compare very unfavourably with men's (around 80 per cent), even allowing for the difference in working hours. This can, as we have seen, cause difficulties for women, if their husbands are unemployed or they are lone mothers and resources are scarce, and may affect their diets. Yet for many women the fact that they have less spending money (which is also influenced by the allocation of resources within families) can have beneficial effects on mortality levels, since they often have less money to buy alcohol and cigarettes.

Second, the domestic division of labour, which means that women not only bear children but also tend to have greater day-to-day responsibility for bringing them up, also has an impact on women's mortality and morbidity and their use of health services. I have already noted how women's health (as well as family health) has benefited enormously from the reductions in family size that have occurred during this century. Frequent pregnancies and large families can pose an enormous direct burden on women's physical health and make it very difficult for them to ensure adequate diets for themselves and their families. Having large numbers of children can also be stressful for women, although there is evidence that the period with young children is stressful for women nowadays even if they have only one (Popay 1992).[15] The gains for women's health from the marked decline in average family sizes during this century are undoubtedly considerable, and have not been offset by the adverse effects of their increased participation in the labour market, which has itself been clearly facilitated by the decline in childbearing. Not only do women generally do safer, less dangerous work than men, but their increased participation in the labour market has helped to increase family resources amongst couples and make poverty less likely. It also improves their psychological health. Analysis of data from the Health and Lifestyle Survey (Bartley et al. 1992) showed that women in full-time and part-time work had better physical and mental health than housewives.

However, whilst the decline in family size has generally been beneficial for women's health, women's greater involvement in childbearing and childrearing in comparison with men is highly pertinent in accounting for reported morbidity that is as high or higher than men's, and women's greater use of health services viewed across the life-span as a whole. Taken together, the data suggest that nowadays women's higher reported morbidity is more a product of different thresholds and standards of illness than of greater ill-health.

Of overriding significance is the fact that women's greater involvement with childbearing and child-rearing means that they tend to be the 'providers, negotiators and mediators' in relation to health maintenance and health care within families and couples: they are expected to secure 'the domestic conditions necessary for the maintenance of health and the recovery from sickness' (Graham 1985: 26), to set standards of diet and discipline and create a culture of health, and to act as go-betweens linking informal and formal health care. This health consciousness is part of what being an effective, competent mother requires. During pregnancy and after childbirth women's health and that of their babies has to be regularly monitored. When this period of close medical supervision is over, women are supposed, as part of their domestic responsibilities, especially if they have no paid or only part-time paid employment, to be the ones who concern themselves with their children's health (and their partners) and to provide much of the informal health care. And when they take their children to doctors they may have an opportunity to raise problems about their own health (many also have contact with doctors of necessity because of contraception, or problems with menstruation or the menopause). At the same time as requiring more contact with the health services, women's obligations as mothers require an attention to health matters that makes it more likely that they will admit to health problems. This health consciousness is likely to persist even when child-rearing is completed, and to extend to the majority of women whether they have had children or not, since they are likely to be socialized into the same expectations and may have similar obligations to elderly parents if not to their own children. Consequently, issues surrounding reproduction and caring directly and indirectly account for much of women's raised contact with health professionals and self-reported morbidity.

This analysis is backed by a range of data. Studies indicate, as I noted in Chapter 1, that much of women's excess level of hospital admissions is due to reproduction; when such conditions are excluded the difference is diminished (Macfarlane 1990). The same also applies to visits to GPs. Studies also generally show a greater willingness by women to report health problems, particularly milder problems, with a number showing that the more severe the illness the smaller the gender difference in self-reports (Nathanson 1977). One study showed that men were more likely than women to rate their symptoms more highly than a clinical observer (MacIntyre 1993). However, whilst this could be taken to suggest that they generally have a lower tolerance level for symptoms of illness and will over-report them, it can equally be read as indicating that women make more accurate assessments of health (fitting the thesis of women's greater responsibility and experience with health and illness). Moreover, the finding is not incompatible with the observation that women are more willing to report symptoms in the first place.

An important issue which needs separate consideration is that of psychological ill-health, since the higher rates of reported psychological morbidity in women, particularly in relation to symptoms of anxiety and depression, have been widely noted, though there is recent, limited evidence of increases in male rates of depression but not female (Shajahan and Cavanagh 1998). It is significant in this connection that women in Britain currently attach more importance to psychological well-being than men (Blaxter 1990: 18), a factor that would contribute to a greater willingness amongst women to report psychological symptoms which has been shown in several studies (Phillips and Segal 1969; Horwitz 1977; Padesky and Hammen 1981). But the issue is not simply one of willingness to report more symptoms, but also of the gendered way in which psychological problems are expressed and the way in which the boundaries of less severe mental disorder have been constructed and are applied. Women who are under stress tend to become anxious and depressed and more readily become 'cases' of mental illness, whereas men under stress, who drink too heavily or become physically or sexually abusive, are less likely to be regarded as mentally disturbed. This is because there is a tendency to focus on their behaviour rather than their mental states, and to assume them to be agents. As a result, when men's conduct is judged to be unacceptable it is more likely to be viewed as delinquent or deviant than as symptomatic of mental illness (Busfield 1996: ch. 6). In contrast, since emotional expression is more normative in women, tension and difficulties are likely to be channelled in this way and states of anxiety and depression are more likely to be identified. Consequently, gender differences in observed psychological morbidity, whilst they almost certainly indicate that women do experience more depression and anxiety, cannot be treated as indicative of real differences in the levels of underlying psychological difficulties.

A final factor requiring consideration is the fact that because women live longer than men and tend to marry men who are older than them, they are more likely in old age to be widowed and end up living on their own. This not only exposes them to the stress of bereavement, but may also leave them socially isolated. They are also more likely to be in poverty (Arber and Ginn 1991). In addition, since proportionately more women survive to older ages, there is to some extent a lower selection for fitness and health than amongst men. This suggests that the observed gender difference in morbidity amongst the elderly is due in part to the fact that many of the less healthy men have already died. However, there may also be some difference in the standards of health set by older men and women. Women may set higher standards of health and lower thresholds of illness and incapacity than men because of the continuing need to fulfil domestic obligations at a time when men have retired.

A number of writers suggest that, even allowing for these tendencies, overall there is almost certainly higher morbidity amongst women than men (Benzeval et al. 1995: 2; Thomas 1995; Nettleton 1995: 176–84). However, I argued in Chapter 1 that the evidence indicates the morbidity levels of men and women are not very dissimilar. The conundrum comes from the fact that we might expect, given their higher mortality, that male rates of morbidity would be significantly higher. In my view, however, there is sufficient evidence of differences in contact with the medical profession, and in willingness to report symptoms as a result of women's typically greater responsibility for health, to make the claim that female morbidity is higher rather suspect.

Conclusion

Whilst material factors are undoubtedly decisive in accounting for the long-term decline in mortality between the eighteenth and twentieth centuries, both material factors and social relations contribute to the class inequalities in health which help to limit the current achievements in longevity. In the case of gender differences, though genetic factors almost certainly play some part, the gender division of labour and the material differences in men's and women's lives it occasions are crucial. Men die younger because they are exposed to more dangerous work (and to a lesser extent leisure) environments, have less healthy lifestyles, and find their paid jobs more stressful. Women's longevity, which was in the past typically curtailed by numerous pregnancies and large families (in situations where resources were scarce), has increased more rapidly than men's (though men's health also benefited from the reduction in family sizes). Women, however, by virtue of their roles as providers, negotiators, and mediators of health, report as many or more symptoms of ill-health as men.

Chapter 4

Health Care in Britain

THE British health care system is dominated by the National Health Service, which came into existence on 5 July 1948 as part of the postwar welfare settlement. The NHS provides publicly funded health services that are available to the whole population. In this respect it offers a service grounded in the principles of universalism, with entitlement to the service based on citizenship, as William Beveridge envisaged in his 1942 Report:

> a comprehensive national health service will ensure that for every citizen there is available whatever medical treatment he requires, in whatever form he requires it, domiciliary or institutional, general, specialist or consultant, and will ensure also the provision of dental, ophthalmic and surgical appliances, nursing and midwifery and rehabilitation after accidents. (1942: para. 427)

This universalism is the hallmark of the NHS and arguably a feature that has contributed to its popularity, since it makes health care a right and incorporates principles of equality and fairness. Universal entitlement to public-sector (in the sense of state-organized) health care on the basis of citizenship contrasts with two main alternatives to state welfare services: entitlement based on labour market status, where those who are employed are eligible for health care, which is usually funded through compulsory insurance; and entitlement based on financial need, where the state funds health care for a residual group of those who cannot afford to purchase it themselves and who are not covered by their employment (Esping-Andersen 1990; Sainsbury 1996: 44–6). Britain is not alone in having a state system of health care that is universal in terms of entitlement (others include Scandinavia, Italy, Spain, Canada, and Brazil), although it is unusual in that the majority of funding comes from taxation rather than compulsory state insurance. The reasons for the fact that a universal national health service was introduced in Britain relatively early (the first in Europe; the Soviet Union had a universal system from 1938) have been a matter of some debate and will be discussed in the next chapter, as will the differences between welfare state regimes.

In this chapter I want to describe the health care system in Britain by setting out where it stands in relation to seven key dimensions: (i) the particular mixture of state versus private sector provision—the so-called public/private mix; (ii) the balance of hospitals versus primary care within the health services; (iii) the degree to which it is dominated by the medical profession; (iv) the extent to which it is committed to the use of science, technology, and biomedicine; (v) the degree to which it is oriented to treating sickness versus maintaining health; (vi) its accessibility; and (vii) its funding arrangements. In each case I point to some of the major changes over time.

The public/private mix in the provision of health care

State or public (the two words are usually used interchangeably) health services, even when they are available to all as a right of citizenship, invariably coexist with private health care which is available as an alternative to those who can afford it—the extent of the private sector varying from country to country. In addition, state health care systems, whatever the basis of entitlement, vary in precisely what they cover (significantly, a decision was made to incorporate mental health services into the NHS when it was set up), and in the extent to which they rely on private-sector services—pharmaceuticals and equipment on the one hand, and private hospitals and doctors on the other.[1]

The contrast made between public and private in such discussions is a complex one and is usually based on a range of criteria. The contrast can be illuminated for our purposes by setting out three ideal typical models of medical care—public, private, and voluntary—and using them as a template for purposes of comparison of the specificities of the health care arrangements in a given society.[2] The ideal typical model of state health care provision is of services to which all are entitled by virtue of citizenship and which are allocated on the basis of medical need rather than ability to pay. In order to accomplish this goal, the services are owned and managed by the state, doctors are salaried employees (necessary to ensure their compliance with the requirements of the system and to keep costs down), and the services are provided 'free at the point of use'—that is, there is no relationship between use and cost to the individual. In contrast, in the ideal typical model of private health services, services are assumed to be based on the principles of the market, with doctors who own their premises acting as self-employed traders in the market (though regulation is typically considered necessary to ensure that only appropriately qualified doctors can practise), and charges are set at levels that the market will bear, patients being charged according to the services they receive. A third ideal type covering the characteristics of charitable/voluntary sector of health care can also be added (where only a public/private contrast is made voluntary provision is placed in the private sector). In this ideal type a charitable body, funded by donations, provides services without charge and the doctor offers the medical services free. The contrast between the three models is set out in Table 4.1. The analysis suggests a number of possible criteria of state provision, including ownership and/or management, entitlement, and funding.

One variation of some importance not captured by these three ideal types is that between private health care, provided by individual practitioners who own their own premises from which they provide services (the classic fee-for-service model), and private health care, where the service is owned and run by someone else, either a providential trust or company on a non-profit-making basis, or a commercial company as a profit-making business. Such arrangements are often necessary when hospitals are needed, since they require major capital investment. Whereas providential groups typically employ doctors on a fee-for-service basis, commercial companies often employ them on a salaried basis in order to keep costs down. A further complexity in the private sector is the development of companies providing health insurance enabling individuals to spread the costs and risks of private health care, again either on a providential or commercial basis. Three different models of private health care need, therefore, to be distinguished; they are set out in Table 4.2 A central feature of both providential and commercial health care is that, as in state medicine, a third party, often with considerable powers, enters the picture and mediates the relationship between practitioner and patient (see Johnson 1972).

The British NHS does not correspond very precisely to the ideal type of state health care except on the issue of entitlement, and is strikingly hybrid in character. The NHS still reflects many of the features of the different components of

Table 4.1 Public, private, and voluntary models of medical care

	Public	Private	Voluntary
Ownership and management	State	Independent practitioner	Charity
Entitlement	Citizenship	Ability to pay	Medical/social need
Cost to user	Free	Fee for service	Free
Doctor's status	Salaried	Self-employed	Honorary
Funding	Taxation	Charges	Donations

Table 4.2 Models of private health care

	Private practitioner	Providential	Commercial
Ownership and management	Individual practitioner	Providential group (non-profit-making)	Commercial company (profit-making)
Entitlement	Ability to pay	Ability to pay/insurance	Ability to pay/insurance
Cost to user	Fee for service	Fee/insurance premium	Fee/insurance premium
Doctor's status	Independent	Independent	Salaried
Funding	Charges	Charges/insurance	Charges/insurance

health care that were taken over when it was established, and the success of doctors in retaining many of the features of practice to which they were committed. Within the NHS, the hospital sector fits most closely to the ideal type of public sector provision. NHS hospitals are publicly owned, managed, and funded, doctors are salaried, services are provided free at the point of use, and funding comes from general taxation. The majority had initially developed as charitable institutions within the voluntary sector, although there were some state-sector municipal general hospitals and mental hospitals (often former Poor Law institutions) and some private nursing homes and small hospitals. When the NHS was set up, all except the private nursing homes were taken into national ownership and the control of central government, though with local management boards (earlier plans had often envisaged they would become municipal hospitals under local government control). From 1990 onwards an increasing number of NHS hospitals took on trust status and the ownership of assets was transferred to the trusts, though still under public ownership and central control.[3]

In contrast, primary care departs quite considerably from the ideal-typical model. Under the 1911 National Insurance Act which made employment status (initially only in certain industries) the basis of entitlement, GP services were available to insured persons through the panel system.[4] When the NHS was established, primary care services were made available to all, initially without direct charge (though limited charging was soon introduced at the primary care level). However, GPs, pharmacists, dentists, and opticians were contracted as 'independent practitioners' to provide NHS services in premises which they continued to own.[5] Instead of being salaried, GPs were initially paid on a capitation basis in terms of the numbers of patients on their lists with a limited fee-for-service element (the same mix that had operated under national insurance arrangements). In the mid-1960s, after further negotiations, a basic allowance for GPs with over 1,000 patients was agreed, introducing what amounts to a salary component in their pay. NHS dentists, in contrast, have largely been paid for on a fee-for-service basis, as have NHS pharmacists and opticians.[6]

Whilst the NHS remains the predominant provider of health services in Britain (accounting for 89 per cent of UK health expenditure in 1991 (Allsop 1995: 74), private health services have continued to operate alongside the NHS since its inception. These take many forms. At the primary care level, NHS GPs (that is, those who are contracted to provide NHS services) were given the freedom to treat private patients. However, private medical practice at the primary care level has never been very significant since the NHS was set up. It has been estimated that 95 per cent of the population had registered with a GP by the end of the first two months of the operation of the NHS (Lindsey 1962), and subsequent registration levels have remained as high as this. Of course patients registered with a NHS GP can also consult a GP on a private basis (either the same or another one). However, the incentives for patients to pay for GP care have usually been small. The majority of GPs decided to join the NHS and to take NHS patients, so patients had access to the same doctors as they would if they paid privately. Some NHS GPs do see patients privately but since access to NHS GPs is generally considered adequate, relatively few pay for GP care and most insurance schemes have not included GP services, though there are signs that commercial companies are trying to expand the market for private general practice.[7]

At the specialist, secondary care level the situation in relation to private practice has been rather different. Most hospital doctors chose to work within the NHS since all the major hospitals were incorporated into it and, very importantly, consultants were allowed to opt for part-time NHS contracts. This enabled them to carry on private practice with both in- and out-patients alongside NHS work—an ideal contractual mix if they could attract private patients, since it meant higher incomes with no loss of job security. Private in-patients could be treated either in 'pay-beds' in NHS hospitals (another residue from pre-NHS days when the voluntary hospitals had fee-paying as well as free patients) or in the small private hospitals or nursing homes which were not taken over into state ownership (most were then run on providential lines). Initially, though potentially lucrative to consultants, the use of private hospital beds was not very extensive and was restricted then as now largely to what is termed 'cold' or 'elective' surgery—that is, operations, often quite minor, that can be planned in advance rather than emergency interventions. For patients the advantages were choice of consultant, a private room with more domestic comforts, and a choice of when to be admitted to hospital, but there were few if any actual medical advantages (and the lack of night-time medical cover and other specialist expertise when problems arise has been a real disadvantage). The disadvantages to NHS users have been the loss from the NHS of medical and nursing staff trained largely at the state's expense, and the subsidizing of pay-beds, as well as the fracturing of the principle of the allocation of health services on the grounds of medical need rather than ability to pay (Higgins 1988).

Private primary and secondary health care, often by NHS doctors, are two areas of private work, the latter more important than the former. A third area is the care provided by a range of specialist health practitioners (mostly not medically qualified) who operate outside the NHS and provide services usually not available or difficult to obtain on the NHS. The list includes psychotherapists, physiotherapists, and specialists in 'alternative' medicine such as reflexologists, hypnotists, chiropractitioners, and osteopaths, who have rarely been found in the NHS contexts, and, to an increasing extent, dentists. Most of these professionals work as private independent practitioners on a fee-for-service basis and their activities correspond closely to the ideal type, private practitioner model. Fourth and finally, there is the expanding sector of private residential nursing care for those needing longer-term care. However, as I noted in Chapter 1, drawing the boundary between health and social care is not easy. In an effort to cut health care costs (provided on a universal basis), there have been enormous pressures to treat longer-term care as social not health care, since social care is provided free only to those in financial need. The consequence has not only been a narrowing of the boundaries of health care but an expansion of private residential care.

Consideration of these four types of private health care is important in illuminating one vital point about the public/private mix of health care in Britain: this it operates not just at the level of service provision but also at the level of the individual user. Whilst the NHS is the dominant provider, more people make occasional use of private health care than one might expect, even if it is only in the form of private physiotherapy or treatment from an osteopath or psychotherapist (if we included over-the-counter medicines there would surely be no exceptions). The extent of this use is partly structured by the availability of NHS services. Where there are weaknesses in NHS provision, private services are more likely to flourish. Dentists, paid largely on a fee-for-service basis within the NHS, have increasingly argued that fees have been inadequate, and many have discontinued NHS work except for children. In some cases, as with chiropractic, and other forms of alternative medicine, NHS work is almost non-existent. On the other hand, even those most ideologically committed to private medicine are unlikely to be able to avoid all contact with the NHS during their lifetime. Many people with private medical insurance still use an NHS GP, and even if they do not, almost everyone who suffers some relatively severe accident or has a serious illness is likely to end up in NHS care (Busfield 1990).[8] This is important because it means we cannot divide the population into private- and public-sector consumers in any simple way: it helps to account for the support for the NHS across social classes, and for the fact the private health care does not confer much in the way of longer-term class advantage in the way that, for instance, private education does.

The analysis of the different components of private health care also provides a framework for examining changes in the overall balance of public and private care since the NHS was established. In the early decades the private sector appeared relatively unimportant. Initially there were round 8,500 pay-beds in NHS hospitals out of a total of 544,000 beds (Webster 1988: 122), and there were about 250 small private hospitals and nursing homes, mostly run by providential associations on a non-profit making basis. Pay-beds declined in number during the 1950s and 1960s, and the 1974–9 Labour Government planned to phase them out altogether. However, from the 1970s onwards a number of factors started to increase the importance of the private sector (notwithstanding Labour's pay-bed policy). On the one hand, the key private-sector actors involved in the provision of private health insurance and of private hospitals began to become more active and more commercial in their operations—a shift accelerated by the neo-liberal philosophies and policies of Conservative administrations between 1979 and 1997. On the other hand, the pressures on the NHS increased as a result of public expenditure concerns generated by the oil crisis, demographic change, and medical innovations (see Chapter 6)—pressures marked most visibly by a concern about waiting lists—and this allowed the private companies to develop private-sector hospital provision and to encourage people to take out private health care insurance. Marked changes in the sector followed: most private medical insurance had been run by providential associations, but from the late 1970s commercial companies and commercial principles began to take a greater hold. For example, in 1978 the British United Provident Association established a new profit-making subsidiary, BUPA Hospitals; it began television advertising in 1979 and doubled its advertising budget between 1979 and 1981 (Griffith and Rayner 1985). This greater commercialism in the private sector, combined with active government support from 1979 onwards, ensured an overall expansion in private health care most visible in the increased numbers covered by private medical insurance.[9] The UK numbers expanded from around 2 million at the beginning of the 1970s to 6.7 million in 1990. This was the peak year, and since then there has been some decline to 5.7 million by 1995 (ONS 1997c: table 8.16). Despite this expansion, private-sector medical care is still largely limited to elective surgery, and insurance coverage is strongly linked to age since around half are covered by company schemes as a result of their employment status (medical insurance is one of their occupational benefits) and many lose their insurance on retirement. It is also related to class, with the middle and upper classes more likely to have private medical insurance than the working classes—in 1995 over 20 per cent of employers, managers, and professionals compared with under 4 per cent of the non-manual groups (ONS 1997b: table 8.4).[10]

The political pressure under Conservative administrations to make greater use of private-sector providers and to privatize some services reflects another important component of the public/private mix in health care. This is the reliance of the NHS on private companies in many different ways: from the building of hospitals to equipment and pharmaceutical companies—a reliance that is continuing under the Labour Government. Of these commercial companies the most important grouping are the pharmaceutical companies, not only in terms of the proportion of the NHS budget spent on drugs but also in terms of their power and influence over the content of medical practice itself (see Chapter 5).

Hospital versus primary care

It is clear from the discussion in the previous section that there is an important institutional divide within the NHS between hospital and primary care—that is, care from a GP or other health professional that may precede contact with specialist doctors (albeit sometimes in their consulting-rooms outside the hospital, or an out-patient clinic) but often does not. Some such divide is typical of advanced Western health care systems, though precisely how it is drawn varies. In Germany, for instance, the key divide is between in-patient hospital care and 'ambulatory care', which includes out-patient services (Moran 1994), whereas in Britain the key distinction is between generalist (primary) and specialist (hospital) care. Health care systems also vary in the importance attached to hospital as opposed to primary or ambulatory care. Western medicine has been characterized by the dominance of hospital-based medicine and Britain follows that pattern, although primary care has been given rather more importance in Britain than in other advanced industrial societies (in the US, for instance, hospital medicine is even more predominant), in large part because of the way in which in Britain access to hospital care is usually mediated by GPs.

The underlying dominance of hospitals over primary care in Britain is most obviously evidenced by the relatively low proportion of resources spent on primary care. Around a quarter of NHS spending is now on primary care (GP, pharmaceutical, dental, and ophthalmic services). The rest goes on hospitals (the largest proportion), community health services, ambulance services, national and regional administration, and some centrally funded services such as research and development costs.[11]

In Britain, hospitals began to emerge as the key locations for medical practice in the second half of the eighteenth century, when a wave of new hospitals were established as charitable institutions on the basis of voluntary subscriptions. They were designed to provide medical care for those of 'middling circumstances' and the respectable poor who could not afford to pay for medical services (though initially they focused on care as much as treatment (Abel-Smith 1964)). Patients tended to be sent there on the advice of their doctor (often as part of their employers' patronage) and received care free of charge (Woodward 1974). But the hospitals were eschewed by the more affluent members of the population who could afford to have their medical services provided at home, and their reputation was not very high. Patients were reluctant to enter them, since the treatments provided were typically very painful and often ineffective. However, in the second half of the nineteenth century the image of the hospital began to change. One important factor was the change in nursing practice. Nursing reforms affected the status of those who worked as nurses, and the hospital's cleanliness and hygiene enhanced their reputation. The regimen of the hospital (including, for instance, the control of alcohol) was itself designed in ways that were intended to facilitate health and might well be considered healthier than the home environment (though there were dangers of infection—specialist fever hospitals were one response to this). The introduction of new treatments and new technologies also helped to change the image of hospitals, with new anaesthetics such as chloroform and antisepsis in surgery of particular significance in the second half of the nineteenth century (Porter 1999: ch. 12).

Hospitals also played a key role in changing the character of medical work. Jewson (1976) has distinguished three phases of medical practice each with its own cosmology. The first, bedside medicine, developed outside the hospital. Here disease was defined in terms of its external and subjective manifestations and was viewed as a disturbance of the integrated totality of the psyche and soma. The practitioner viewed the patient as a person and adopted an active, therapeutic role through the heavy applications of heroic remedies (blood-letting was a common treatment). However, during the early decades of the nineteenth century bedside medicine was replaced by a new cosmology that emerged in the context of the hospital—hospital medicine. In this form of medicine the focus was on organic lesions within the body, with anatomy increasingly important as the basis of medical knowledge; the patient was viewed as a case; and the major task was that of the diagnosis and classification of disease. Jewson suggests that from the middle of the nineteenth century a third type of medicine began to emerge, laboratory medicine, with disease viewed as a biochemical process, the patient as but a complex of cells, and the medical task being primarily that of analysis and explanation. In his view both hospital and laboratory medicine, which are both forms of what is now usually called biomedicine (i.e. medicine that focuses on the body), shifted the focus away from the person and instead treated patients more as things and objects, so distancing the doctor from the patient.

Since the development of hospitals in the first half of the eighteenth century, doctors who worked in them (at first as honorary physicians who received no pay) have tended to have higher status than other doctors (those from higher-status backgrounds were in a better position to secure the post of honorary physician, which enhanced their status and could give them access to wealthy clients in their private practice outside the hospital). This position in the medical hierarchy was further strengthened by the development of specialist expertise (itself facilitated by hospital work), which meant that more generalist doctors might have to refer their most difficult cases to hospital doctors (even though they often feared losing their subsequent custom). The expertise of hospital doctors and the status that accrued to it was recognized and consolidated through membership of the Royal Colleges. Once this position was secured, the competition between specialists and generalists was regulated by the decision that access to specialists would be via the general practitioners (Abel-Smith 1964)—a very important feature of medical practice in Britain, since it made GPs the gatekeepers of specialist medicine and provided a means whereby GPs could limit the demands on specialist medicine to 'reasonable' levels (though GPs' ideas as to when it is reasonable to refer a patient to a specialist vary, as do their levels of specialist referral (Coulter, 1992); however, they can usually make more informed decisions than patients, and their gatekeeping role has been very important in helping to keep NHS costs down).

Childbirth provides an example of the increasing strength of the pro-hospital ideology in the twentieth century, and has been seen by many as evidence of the growing influence of the medial profession. Prior to the Second World War most births took place at home, with women often attended by a midwife rather than a doctor, though the proportion of hospital births was already rising (in 1927, 15 per cent of births took place in hospital; by 1937 the figure was 35 per cent). Concern about continuing high levels of maternal (and infant) mortality were used to argue that hospital deliveries were safer, as they offered the possibility of techniques for inducing labour, Caesareans, and drugs and oxygen as necessary. By 1957 two-thirds (65 per cent) of births were occurring in hospital, a figure that had risen to 91 per cent by 1972 (Oakley 1983; 1986) and is now even higher.

Three subsequent changes have challenged the pre-eminence of hospital-based medicine in recent decades. One has been the sharp decline in the lengths of stay of patients admitted to hospital and the growth of day surgery. These changes are partly due to new technologies which allow for less invasive interventions (keyhole surgery is a recent example) and therefore a shorter period of recovery, partly to changing ideas about the importance of getting patients 'back on their feet' as soon as possible to aid recovery, and partly to the costs of providing lengthy hospital stays (for example, whereas most women give birth in hospital, their stays are now typically very short). The mean duration of stay in NHS hospitals in acute wards has declined from 14.5 days in 1961 to 7.7 in 1981 and to 5.4 in 1995–6 (CSO 1971: table 39; ONS 1997c: table 8.12) and there has been a rapid growth of day surgery (from 24 per cent of all surgery in 1982 to 34 per cent in 1990 (Allsop 1995: 82)). The reduction in lengths of stay has meant that far fewer hospital beds are needed, though new forms of treatment, including new forms of surgery, do act as something of a counter-pressure. From the initial 544,000 NHS beds the number had fallen to around 256,000 by 1997–8.[12]

The second change is the power that is increasingly being given to GPs to make decisions about what hospital treatment is needed. In Britain, as I have noted, GPs have long had an important role as the gatekeepers to hospital care, making decisions as to whether to refer a patient to a specialist or not. However, following the 1990 NHS and Community Care Act their role as fundholders purchasing elective surgery and some other specialist services has given them an important say in deciding what specialist treatments are to be made available, and this role is being expanded by the Labour Government.[13] It is now introducing primary care commissioning using locally based primary care groups covering areas coterminous with local authorities, and these groups are likely to be purchasing a wider range of services than GP fundholders (Secretary of State for Health 1997).[14]

The third challenge to the power of hospitals has been the growth of community care. This is a very loose, imprecise term, but is mainly used to refer to the provision of a range of facilities for those with chronic problems that do not involve in-patient hospital care. Particularly widely used in the context of mental health services where it tended initially to mean services for those with chronic mental health problems outside the framework of the old asylums and mental hospitals (Busfield 1986: ch. 10), it has also been extensively used in relation to care for the elderly and those with physical or mental incapacities. In many respects those with chronic problems, which are very unlikely to be amenable to medical treatment, are precisely the groups that have threatened the medical character of hospitals, and to that extent community care arguably strengthens rather than undermines the domination of hospitals. Yet at the same time the growth of community care ensures that much health care takes place outside the framework of hospitals and is not subordinate to them. Some of this care, as I noted earlier, is being transferred from health to social services; much involves collaboration between the two.

Medical dominance

Health services vary in the extent to which doctors are the all-powerful actors. In some services their expertise and training ensures that they are treated as gods who make all the key decisions; in others they have a more humble role as the employees and servants of more powerful masters (theoretical ideas about medical power are examined in the next chapter). How powerful are doctors within the NHS? Does the fact that doctors operate within a state system of health care diminish their importance? Certainly many have argued that it does. Here is what Rudolf Klein has to say discussing the situation of the medical profession in the early years of the NHS, and linking the extent of medical power to the arenas in which doctors operate:

> What this would suggest is that the power of the medical profession is in an inverse relationship to the size of the stage on which a specific health care issue is fought out. When the stage widens to bring in actors who normally play no part in the health care arena strictly defined—when the Treasury and the Cabinet become involved—then the ability of the medical profession to get its own way diminishes. Once the issue is defined as that of financial control—when it is seen, in other words, as an issue revolving around national economic strategy rather than health care considerations—the medical profession simply becomes a small battalion facing heavyweight armies. Conversely, the medical profession's influence expands as the stage narrows: becoming in effect total when health care reaches the stage of a duet between doctor and patient. (1995: 50–1)

We need, as Klein suggests, to examine the different arenas in which doctors can exercise power. I want to consider three: their power over their patients; their power within the health care division of labour—that is, the division of different health care tasks between different occupational groups involved in health care; and their power over the structure and organization of the health services in which they operate. In each case, as we shall see, the extent of medical power is influenced by the social and economic context of their work, as Klein's analysis indicates, but this context does not operate in the same way in each arena.

Sickness and illness increase vulnerability, and doctors, as persons with expertise in the care and treatment of illness, have extensive power over their patients. It has been argued, however, that in private practice, despite the perceived attractions for doctors of freedom and autonomy, medical power is somewhat diminished, since the patients are the paymasters and the doctors are dependent on them for their income (this may particularly give more affluent, higher-status patients more power, as doctors are likely to be keen to keep them as patients). Certainly there is evidence that in private practice doctors adopt a more personal approach in dealing with their patients who are more likely to question the competence of the practitioner (Silverman 1987: ch. 5). Moreover, clinical decisions may be constrained by the patient's capacity to pay (the patient may not be able to afford the preferred treatment, or the doctor may be influenced consciously or unconsciously in deciding what to do by the patient's resources as in cases of 'unnecessary treatment'—see Chapter 6). Conversely, state medicine arguably increases doctors' power over their patients, since patients are recipients of state welfare which may make them feel dependent. However, again the class dimension is significant: when patients are middle-class and where entitlement is more of a right and is not seen as a mark of poverty this perception is probably less common—which is one of the benefits of universal state provision.

Doctors' power within the health care division of labour has typically been extensive and this applies in Britain as in other advanced Western countries. Doctors have tended to be at the top of the health care hierarchy, with other care professionals playing a subordinate role, as some of the current terminology reflects—for instance, the term 'paramedical professions'. This hierarchy has been particularly manifest in hospitals where senior doctors have been treated with deference and respect. Historically nurses have been subordinate to doctors and have done the lower-status, more routine, 'dirtier' types of work. Some professional groups such as midwives have had a less obviously subordinate role to doctors, but over time their powers have been whittled away (Donnison 1977). However, some of the newer health care professionals are managing to secure some independence and autonomy—psychologists are one example—and others, for varying reasons, are increasing their power and so represent a challenge to medicine (Gabe et al. 1994). One example is the development of a group of advanced nursing practitioners with more specialist expertise and limited powers of prescribing. Again the degree of medical power is influenced by the social and economic context of their work. Where doctors are in private practice they can employ other health professionals in a subordinate role; where they work in the state system they may have to accept that other professionals may be given more power than they would choose. Whether doctors do have to accept such curtailments or not depends on their power within that organizational context—the third arena where doctors' power needs to be examined.

Historically, even where doctors have not owned the health services in which they have operated, they have played a crucial role in determining the content of medical work and in the management of health institutions. For instance, when the NHS was established doctors were key figures on the hospital management committees and on the executive boards which oversaw the family doctor services, in each case supported by health service administrators, just as they had been key figures in the voluntary hospital management committee and insurance committee boards which the new groups replaced (Webster 1988: 274–82). These management structures typically encouraged consensual management, and the medical influence was considerable. However, during the Conservative administrations from 1979 to 1997 there was a shift from consensus management to a new managerialism which was held to be more consistent with the business ethos that was to imbue the NHS. In 1983 Roy Griffiths, the managing director of Sainsbury, was asked to report on management in the NHS. His brief, influential report (DHSS 1983) called for the appointment of a single general manager for each health service body, who need not be medically qualified and who was to manage the services on business lines in the interests of effectiveness. His recommendations were quickly adopted, but there is evidence that initially the new breed of managers who replaced the health service administrators did not succeed in challenging medical power to any great extent, doctors continuing, for example, to be well represented on the key decision making bodies (Hunter 1994).

The introduction of the internal market in 1990, with the requirement of setting contracts between purchasers and providers, considerably enhanced the power of managers and began seriously to challenge that of consultants (Hunter 1994). The tight limits on budgets set constraints on the number and type of operations that could be carried out and increased the demands for 'evidence-based practice', that is, the use of treatments that have been shown through scientific research, not clinical belief, to be effective (see Chapter 6). In addition, management committees were streamlined so that a typical committee might contain only one doctor. Nonetheless doctors have retained a fair degree of power within the restructured NHS, and the threatened 'proletarianization' of the profession (a term invoked to indicate a loss of control over the conditions of their work and far greater scrutiny of their activity) has not really occurred (Hunter 1994). A major reason has been doctors' continuing control over the content of medical work. They still make the key clinical decisions about patients, deciding what treatments are most appropriate, and they still shape the content and direction of what is constituted as medical knowledge contributing to the shaping of public demand for the provision of particular service. Consequently, though they may operate within tight economic constraints and face greater pressure to show the effectiveness of their interventions, they still have considerable power to shape the character of the NHS. There is little sign that their dominance is under very serious threat. The Labour Government's reforms of the NHS emphasize cooperation within the service rather than competition, and look likely to reaffirm medical power though, as mentioned earlier, the power of general practitioners may be strengthened at the expense of hospital doctors.

Science, technology, and biomedicine

Analytically separate from the power of the medical profession and the degree of dominance of hospital care within a health system, though related to both, is the extent of reliance on science, technology, and biomedicine. Western health care systems make considerable use of, and are partly shaped by, science and technology and give greatest weight to health care in the form of biomedicine—that is, medicine shaped by concern with the body and the biological sciences.[15] Various types of alternative, more holistic forms of medicine and health care are largely excluded from the NHS and have a relatively small part to play in the overall range of health services. Of course, as Jewson's (1976) analysis indicates, precisely which science is most influential varies over time, with a shift from the dominance of anatomy in the early nineteenth century through to chemistry and biochemistry. At present genetics has become particularly influential. However, there is often a discrepancy between the ideological commitment to science and technology within biomedicine and the reality of the commitment to scientific principles in the day-to-day context of clinical practice.[16] Whilst scientific laboratory research requires careful experimentation comparing groups following agreed scientific standards, clinical work with patients usually requires a more pragmatic, less scientific approach that focuses on the individual. Nonetheless there is little doubt that biomedicine dominates the health care services in Britain and that the services make extensive use of new advances in science and technology, though not as extensive as in, say, the US, and some work is at the forefront of those advances.

In Britain the heavy dependence of health care on science, technology, and biomedicine is most visible in the hospital sector, where they have their roots. Both science and new technologies have had a major impact, especially in recent years, on diagnosis, on techniques of surgery, on the monitoring of patients whilst they are in hospital, and on the use of drugs. X-rays have been a major diagnostic tool since the 1920s (Howell 1995), as has the taking of small samples of tissues or bodily fluids and examining them and testing them in order to identify illnesses. To these techniques, which have now been enhanced and improved, have been added new instruments for seeing the body and making the formerly invisible, visible, including notably CAT (computerized axial tomography) or CT scanners and MRI (magnetic resonance imaging), which provide ways of seeing the body in a three dimensional space. In addition, the harnessing of optical fibre technology has enabled the inspection of inner spaces within the body as in procedures such as endoscopy and broncheoscopy. Together these technologies have helped to transform the 'medical gaze'

(Foucault 1973). At the same time surgery has been transformed, particularly through the harnessing of optical fibre technology, which has enabled the development of keyhole surgery techniques in which surgeons can see inside the body and observe their own surgical interventions, via images relayed to them on screens. Optical fibres also enable lasers to be directed at places within the body for therapeutic purposes without the need for large incisions.

The monitoring of patients in hospital has also been revolutionized by new technologies including electrocardigographs (first developed as early as 1903) to monitor heart functioning, ultrasound to monitor pregnancies, and instruments that monitor brain function. So, too, have a range of surgical techniques, notably transplants, such as heart, lung, and kidney transplants (Porter 1999: 618–23). Though it has not yet had much impact on treatment, work in genetics is a very significant area of medical research and the possibilities of gene therapies are being widely discussed. The identification of genetic risk is already becoming the rationale for some medical interventions, as when a woman genetically at risk of breast cancer has a radical mastectomy for prophylactic purposes.

Equally important to the character of medical practice has been the use of science in the development of new drugs. Drugs play a central role in contemporary medicine, including hospital medicine, helping to sustain and legitimate the biomedical orientation of much health care and the power of the medical profession (see Chapter 5). The pharmaceutical industry, which is global in scope (many of the world's largest companies are pharmaceutical companies) and highly commercial in character, wields enormous power (Abraham 1995). In 1995 some 520 million prescriptions were dispensed in Britain, an average of nearly nine for every man, woman, and child. This level is two-fifths more than in 1981; in 1971 the average number of prescriptions was only just over five per person (ONS 1997c: 145).

Drugs are even more crucial within general practice than in hospital medicine (they currently account for nearly 50 per cent of all primary care spending and 80 per cent of all prescriptions (Davis 1997)). Drugs are the most visible marker of the deployment of science at the primary care level, which is generally characterized by much lower level technology than hospital work. In Britain most of the more sophisticated screening is carried out in hospital contexts (an arrangement that helps to keep costs down). However, GPs do make considerable use of some screening techniques (e.g. for cervical cancer) and blood pressure with or without the aid of laboratory services. The notable area of new technological development in primary care is in the use of information technology, in relation both to record keeping and to access to research findings, and most GPs now use personal computers. The use of IT in these ways also applies to hospital settings, though there have been major problems arising from the implementation of IT programmes and networking in hospitals, with one or two spectacular failures.

Although these new developments in science and technology have considerable potential benefit, there are dangers. One area of danger lies in the reluctance to assess very thoroughly the precise range of the effectiveness of particular procedures and interventions and the overuse of sophisticated technology, issues to which I return in Chapter 6. But there are other concerns. First, medicine's reliance on science and technology encourages an emphasis on the importance of the natural sciences and the belief that there must be a 'technological fix' for any health problem. As a result science (which invariably means the natural sciences) and technology are given primacy at the expense of psychological and social sciences, though the latter may be especially important to disease prevention and can also play a very important role in recovery. Second, it means that considerable prestige accrues to those who are seen to be at the forefront of medical advances in bioscience and technology, especially if they are dealing with life-threatening illnesses. Consequently doctors are encouraged to work in areas where there are potential scientific gains, whether or not these are the fields of most pressing health need. One instance is the lack of interest in the care of the terminally ill for whom there is no prospect of cure. The need to ease the pain and suffering of such patients has lead to the growth of the hospice movement outside the framework of hospitals and standard bio-medicine.[17] Third, medicine's commitment to the use of science and technology accounts for a major part of the increasing costs of medical care (see Chapter 6). By and large the new medical technologies, including new drugs, are very expensive, and though the cost of the new technology may decline a little once it is established and used more widely, this is often compensated for by enhanced specifications. As a result, as with personal computers, instead of prices falling they remain around the same level but the new machinery or the new variant of a drug can do rather more. Clearly the new technologies potentially offer considerable gains which can justify the increased costs, but it is essential that they be used only when needed and when they can be of value, otherwise costs increase yet there is little gain for patients.

Medicine's reliance on science and technology can, as I have already suggested, be linked to its efforts to secure its status as a profession and to obtain powers for its own activities that are denied to other groups of healers—an issue discussed more fully in the next chapter. Science and technology are the basis of its claims to special expertise, and one of the distinctive features of medicine as opposed to other forms of healing. As Parsons puts it, one of the obligations placed on doctors is 'to acquire and use high technical competence in "medical science" and the techniques based upon it' (1951: 447).

Treating sickness versus maintaining health

René Dubos makes a contrast between two fundamental attitudes to medicine and health care: one associated with the goddess Hygeia, the other with the goddess Panacea. Hygeia was concerned with the prevention of disease and the maintenance of health: 'She symbolized the belief that men would remain healthy if they lived wisely, within the golden rule, and according to the laws of reason'; Panacea, who specialized in the knowledge of drugs, focused on curing disease: 'She symbolized the belief that ailments can be cured by skilful use of the proper kinds of substances derived either from plants or from the earth' (Dubos 1968: 79).

In Britain, as in other advanced Western societies, the health care system is overridingly oriented towards curing sickness rather than maintaining health. In terms of its activities and spending the National Health Service would be more accurately described as a National Sickness Service or a National Illness Service. However, in exploring this area we need to differentiate a number of types of preventive work, each with its own trajectory. First, there is *public health medicine*; this is typified by the influential and important work concerning public hygiene and sanitation, especially in relation to infectious illnesses in the nineteenth century, which continues, for instance, in the ongoing work on the safety of food by environmental health officers, but is not restricted to infectious illnesses: the regulation of smoking in public places provides a twentieth-century example of public health work in relation to non-infectious illnesses. This type of work, unlike clinical medicine, is first and foremost concerned with effecting societal-level changes to improve the health of the population rather than focusing on individuals, and has declined in importance in the twentieth century.

Second, there is *health promotion*. This is the type of preventive work that has become especially common in the second half of the twentieth century. Its focus is primarily the health-related behaviours considered in Chapter 2, and though often grounded in epidemiological studies of populations and groups and directed towards changing the behaviour of populations, is largely individually oriented. Its strategies seek to change individuals, typically focusing on individual 'knowledge, attitudes and behaviour'.

Third, there is what I call *clinical prevention*: for instance, the inoculation and screening programmes largely carried out in clinical contexts, but also the use of drugs primarily on preventive grounds, as in the use of Tamoxifen to prevent breast cancer in high-risk women, which has recently aroused some controversy, or the use of hormone replacement therapy for preventive purposes. Again this type of medicine, though it may target populations, involves action at the individual level. Like health promotion, it is almost certainly on the increase. The three types of preventive work are set out in Table 4.3.

Armstrong (1995) groups different types of preventive work together under the broad label, derived from Foucault, of 'surveillance medicine'. He suggests that preventive work blurs the distinction between health and illness and that, in focusing of the precursors of illness—the risk factors—it involves a tight surveillance and control of all aspects of individuals' everyday lives. Other writers have talked instead of 'the new public health' (Nettleton 1995: ch. 9) which they see as spreading medicine's tentacles into all areas of life. I want, however, to make a clear distinction between the three, since they have different proponents and differing financial implications. They also raise very different issues about social control since, whereas health promotion and clinical prevention focus on the individual level, public health focuses primarily on changes at the societal level. The current situation is, therefore, marked by two features: the decline of public health medicine since the nineteenth century (notwithstanding the contrary claims of some writers) and the relatively minor role played by all three types of preventive work within the NHS. How do we account for this situation?

The decline of public health medicine is due to a number of factors. In the first place, the decline of infectious illness as causes of death reduced the public pressure for public health directed at populations and groups rather than individuals, and there have been fewer people articulating demands for public health work.[18] Significantly the BSE scandal has highlighted some of the deficiencies of contemporary public health provision. Second, medicine has largely developed as a profession centred on the care and treatment of sick individuals, who were motivated by their pain and suffering to seek help for

Table 4.3 Types of preventive medicine

Type of preventive medicine	Key characteristics	Examples
Public health	Focuses on societal level changes to improve the population's health	Improved sewerage systems in towns; food hygiene regulations
Health promotion	Focuses on encouraging individuals to change their behaviour	Campaigns about the dangers of excessive drinking, drugs, etc.
Clinical prevention	Individually directed clinical procedures for preventive purposes	Inoculation, vaccination, screening

their problems, and medical activities and medical knowledge have been structured around this clinical work. The collective orientation required for public health medicine is not encouraged by individually-oriented medical practice, which is organized around the care and treatment of particular patients. And third, and related to this, there is potential rivalry and conflicts of interest between public health and clinical medicine, and clinical medicine as the more powerful group has been able, where it has felt threatened, to constrain and limit public health medicine (Lewis 1986). Public health medicine is only likely to have much force if it is embedded in adequate organizational structures and given adequate powers. We can see the importance of institutional structures and arrangements if we look at the history of public health medicine in the NHS.

During the first half of the twentieth century a less clear organizational distinction could be made between public health medicine, health promotion, and clinical prevention. All three were largely in the hands of local authorities under the management of Medical Officers of Health (MOH). The work of local health authorities (LHA) encompassed a range of activities, including the work of municipal hospitals (whose numbers expanded in the 1930s as they were transferred from poor law authorities), maternity and child welfare clinics, ambulance services, school health services, and the work of district nurses and health visitors, as well as disease control and public hygiene. Consequently the work of local health authorities was quite extensive, although the hostility between GPs and MOHs helped to constrain its impact. Moreover, when the NHS was set up, although LHAs continued in existence as one of the three strands of the NHS alongside family practitioner and hospital services, the range of their services was reduced (most obviously the municipal hospitals disappeared from their control) and the MOHs' powers were more restricted than they had been in the nineteenth century.

The 1974 NHS reorganization, the first major reorganization, which attempted to integrate the three strands, made significant changes which further reduced the importance of public health work. It turned MOHs into District Community Physicians (DCP), linking them into the new structure at area level, and transformed some local authority services, such as district nursing and school health services, into community health services. At the same time it left responsibility for some public health matters (for instance, the inspection of premises where food is prepared) with local authorities but entirely outside the NHS, and without the guidance of MOHs, although DCPs could be consulted on such matters. With the 1990 division between purchasers and providers, DCPs ended up in health authorities whose work was concentrated on the purchasing side, whilst community health services took on trust status (either on their own or as part of larger trusts). Overall there are comparatively few

DCPs in the NHS, and increasingly their time is taken up by issues of commissioning health services and with work on rationing criteria and priority setting amongst treatments for those who are already sick rather than doing public health work. The disappearance of the MOHs from the NHS is of considerable importance. Whilst there are those engaged with public health work outside the NHS—safety officers and environmental health inspectors, mainly employed by local authorities, as well as the health and safety at work inspectorate—the public health mentality has largely disappeared from the NHS and preventive work has become a matter of often ineffective health promotion and increasingly expensive clinical prevention.

To argue the case for more public health work is not to dismiss the value of treating sickness. Whilst McKeown's analysis suggests that medicine may have made rather little contribution to long-term declines in the death rate, its contribution in the second half of this century has been rather greater (see Chapter 2), and clinical services certainly relieve pain and suffering. Yet public health work, merits a larger place in health work since the potential health gains are so enormous.[19]

Accessibility

Having health care that is accessible to all members of a society is regarded by many as an essential component of human welfare and of citizenship—a human right that is a *sine qua non* of a just and fair society. Yet the ideal has never been completely achieved. Arguably the British NHS has moved closer than many health care services to providing a highly accessible service by introducing a system based on citizenship, but access is far from prefect and is arguably deteriorating in certain respects, at least in part because some services such as dentistry are becoming harder to obtain on the NHS. Indeed, for a service to be available, and readily available, on the NHS is a precondition of accessibility, and is the area where there is greater cause for concern. Consequently, levels of service provision are a major factor to take into account when considering accessibility. It has long been noted, for example, that the attitudes of local NHS consultants to abortion vary: in some areas it is almost impossible to obtain an NHS abortion. With moves towards priority-setting, which is at present usually determined on a local basis, access to some services may be severely restricted (this matter is discussed further in Chapter 6).

It is also important to note when considering accessibility that some people in Britain are not eligible for NHS services. Entitlement is based on UK citizenship, and reciprocal arrangements are in place with European Union countries to give all EU citizens in the UK access to NHS services. However, non-EU citizens have to pay for NHS services. Consequently, individuals such as asylum seekers, whose status as UK citizens has not been accepted, are not eligible for NHS services. In addition, there is no requirement on GPs to accept homeless individuals on their registers; some make special efforts to provide services for the homeless, others do not.

Apart from issues of the range of service provision and eligibility, which I discuss in Chapter 6, four types of accessibility need to be considered: financial, temporal, geographical, and cultural. Financial accessibility has been the ideological cornerstone of the NHS, which was founded on universal entitlement to the service, and no charges were initially required for any service. However, this principle was very quickly breached with the decision by the Labour Government in 1949 to take powers to introduce a one-shilling prescription charge after concern at the expanding cost of the NHS. In the event charges were not actually introduced until 1951, when the Labour Government, in an effort to limit NHS expenditure, introduced charges for dental and ophthalmic services leading to the resignation of Aneurin Bevan, the Minister of Health who had overseen the introduction of the NHS. The following year the new Conservative administration decided to impose the shilling charge for a prescription. However, the contribution of charges to the cost of the NHS remained at a very low level until the 1980s—it was only 2 per cent in 1978–9 (Royal Commission on the NHS, 1979: table E11). Since then prescription charges have been sharply increased well beyond the rate of inflation (children, the elderly, those needing long-term medication, and those in receipt of income support are exempt from charges). In addition, charges were introduced for eye tests and dental check-ups in 1989 and charges for dental work have been increased significantly (though children, pregnant women, and pensioners are still exempt). Nonetheless, though the proportion of expenditure from charges was about 6 per cent by 1992 (Allsop 1995: 74) it has since declined and is still a relatively low figure. The impact of these charges on accessibility is debated. Conservative administrations in the 1980s frequently pointed out that a very high percentage of NHS prescriptions were dispensed free of charge (now 84 per cent), but those who are exempt have more prescriptions per head than those who are not (as they tend to be groups whose health is poorer), so the proportion of the population who are exempt is actually rather lower. The new Labour Government admitted early on that it had not ruled out making hotel charges for hospital stays in its review of the NHS, but so far it has not decided to introduce them (and the controversy over the early cut in single-parent benefit has made this less likely). The problem is, of course, the expanding cost of health care in a situation where increases in taxation are seen as politically unacceptable (see Chapter 6).

Temporal accessibility needs to be distinguished from financial accessibility, since although there may be no financial barrier to a service it may still not be available when a person needs it. Certainly there are many instances where mortality is reduced if treatment occurs early, as with certain cancers, and doctors have long stressed the value of early treatment. But this is not true of all conditions, not least because in many cases recovery may be spontaneous or a condition may be stable over a long period of time. Having to wait for treatment is not therefore necessarily harmful. In Britain the advent of appointment systems in GP surgeries in contrast to patients simply turning up and waiting as long as necessary has often meant waiting a day or two (often longer) in getting to see a GP, which can be a source of dissatisfaction (though arguably preferable to long queues), but since most GPs have emergency appointments it is not considered to have affected health outcomes adversely. The situation with hospitals is rather different. Waiting-lists for many operations are common (with some people having to wait eighteen months or more), and there can be waits of three or four hours or even longer for treatment in accident and emergency departments.[20] Whilst some of these waits may do little long-term harm, others do, and waiting may also cause anxiety and leave patients in pain and is one of the areas where the NHS is currently least successful. However, it is important to remember that waiting-lists are generated by medical decisions and give no reliable guide to the level of unmet need. Waiting-lists, undesirable though they are, also provide a form of implicit rationing device that serves to keep hospital costs down (see Chapter 6).

Geographical accessibility has two dimensions: the evenness of the distribution of health services in terms of quality and quantity across the country and the specific location of services. The poor overall distribution of health services was one of the main complaints about health services prior to the introduction of the NHS (Eckstein 1958), but once it was set up the issue received little attention during the first decade (Webster 1988: 292), though some incentives and controls were introduced to influence the distribution of GPs. Doctors wishing to move were not allowed to practice in 'over-doctored' areas and received extra payments for working in areas with relatively few doctors (in some rural areas where pharmaceutical services were poor they were also allowed to dispense medicines, which increased their incomes). Whilst regulations on the distribution of GPs have improved the access of those in regionally under-provided areas (though they are still somewhat concentrated in more middle class areas), two further changes have affected accessibility: the shift in GP work from the home to the surgery and the increase in the average size of GP practices.

Medicine provided at home was long the preferred model of the affluent members of the community, while those with fewer resources often relied on potions and remedies bought in the market place; or in cases of extreme need they might be visited on a charitable basis by a official doctor or an unlicensed healer. In the nineteenth century charitable dispensaries provided an important alternative for the poorer sections of the community, but licensed healers continued to practice largely in people's homes. Under the arrangements of the 1911 National Insurance Scheme panel doctors practised from surgeries which patients had to visit, though if they were severely ill they would be visited at home. With the establishment of the NHS the surgery increasingly became the main location for GP work and the amount of home visiting has declined steadily. Whereas 22 per cent of consultations still occurred at home in 1971 only 9 per cent did by 1996 (ONS 1998b: table 8.15), though home visits, usually from a deputizing service, are still significant at night, as well as for those aged 75 or over, where 27 per cent of GP consultations take place at home (ONS 1998b: table 8.22). This shift has meant more of a change for the middle and upper than the working classes, since it was the former who were more likely to have doctors visit at home. However, since the middle and upper classes tend to have better access to private means of transport, the shift has not seriously diminished their access to medical care. For the working classes, particularly women and older people, the reduction in home visits may well have made matters worse, since there can be significant transport difficulties.

A second change that has relevance for the geographical distribution of doctors and geographical access is the increasing shift away from single- or two-person GP practices to ones of five, six, seven, or even more GPs (in 1952 almost 50 per cent of GPs were single-handed; in 1990 fewer than 10 per cent were, and almost 60 per cent of practices contained four doctors or more). This tendency has been counterbalanced a little by the reduction in the average size of GP lists (from 2,150 in 1980 to 1,900 in 1990 (Allsop 1995: 200)) and overall there are now more GPs, though there are some concerns about current levels of recruitment. Nonetheless, the increasing concentration of doctors in larger practices has generally meant a greater geographical concentration of GP services, which also creates problems of access for those without private transport, especially in rural areas. The evidence indicates that larger practices tend to be better—they attract better-qualified doctors and can provide better facilities and support staff—but the transport difficulties for some patients, particularly the elderly, need more attention than they usually receive.

The NHS has also had an impact on the geographical distribution of hospitals over the longer term. When it was set up it simply took over existing hospital stock and no new hospitals were built, so that the distribution of hospitals reflected historical contingencies. In 1962 the Hospital Plan (Ministry of Health 1962) set out for the first time clear norms of hospital provision which regions were to follow when developing their services and capital began to be made available for new hospitals. The Hospital Plan also argued the case for district general hospitals—single centres of excellence with some 600–800 beds for each health district serving a population of around 100,000–150,000—a model that provided the case for some concentration and rationalization of services; however, during the 1970s the plan was modified because of the costs and inconvenience to patients.

Again, however, the period of Conservative governments since 1979 proved to be a period of major change. Their focus on cost-effectiveness combined with the development of new, sophisticated, and very expensive technologies, such as magnetic resonance imaging scanners, once more encouraged the view that some hospital services had to be concentrated in centres of excellence if they were to be of high quality—an argument that has been given weight by studies which show that in some areas of medicine such as cancer treatment, patients treated by specialist cancer surgeons have a better chance of survival than those treated by general surgeons. It was better to have one centre of excellence than two or three less specialized facilities, particularly where very sophisticated techniques and specialist expertise were required. Hence the closure of various accident and emergency services and the closing down of cancer units at some hospitals and their relocation to others, a policy that generated greatest opposition in London. This concentration increases problems of access, including the access of visitors who provide important moral support for patients, particularly in a situation where public transport has deteriorated as it has over the past twenty years. The problem is, of course, that the potential medical gains—which may only be for a few people, though very crucial to them—and the transport difficulties are incommensurate. Those with private transport often only see the medical gains (though some have argued that they are smaller than might be thought or even non-existent); others see very clearly what a significant impact the difficulties of access can have for patients and their families and friends. Many, however, would accept that where concentrating specialist facilities improves outcomes this has in the end to override the other considerations.

Cultural accessibility is the fourth dimension of accessibility. A medical service which deters individuals because it is not, in the current jargon, 'user-friendly' also creates considerable problems and undermines accessibility. One of the key issues is the adequacy of communication between doctor and patient. Where communication is poor, patients find it difficult to say what concerns them and feel reluctant to make use of the services, a problem that can be exacerbated by the bio-medical focus on the body and the lack of interest in patients' experiences of illness. In addition, their problems will be more likely to be misdiagnosed by the doctor. Here the dimensions of age, class, gender, and ethnicity are particularly important, since differences between practitioner and patient on these dimensions can lead to misunderstandings. A range of studies point to the problems of communication between doctor and patient, problems that can mean that those in disadvantaged groups are less likely to get the treatment and care they need.

The extent to which these different aspects of accessibility underpin class differences in the use of the NHS has been a matter for debate. There is some evidence of greater use of services by those in the manual than the non-manual classes. In 1996, for example, 14 per cent of males in the manual classes had visited a GP in the previous 14 days against 13 per cent in the non-manual groups; amongst women the figures were 20 per cent and 17 per cent respectively (ONS 1998b: table 8.24). However, interpretations of such data have differed markedly. Le Grand (1982) argued that the working classes do not use the NHS relative to need as much as the middle classes, and pointed to factors such as the distribution of medical facilities, transport difficulties, and greater problems in taking time off work to visit the doctor. Others have contended that any greater use by the manual classes is in line with (self-assessed) health differences and that there is close to equality of access in terms of need (Collins and Klein 1980).

However, a range of studies dealing with specific services do indicate important class differences in service use, with the working classes typically making less use of these specific services. There is, for instance, evidence that more disadvantaged groups make less use of preventive services such as general health check-ups, screening, immunization, antenatal care, and birth control services. There is also some evidence that GP consultations are marginally longer with middle- than with working-class patients, and referral rates to specialist care per consultation are also higher. Benzeval et al., concluding their summary of the data, note that too little is known about whether access to the NHS matches need, and contend: 'The clear implication is that the NHS should devote more effort to assessing the true extent of inequalities in access to care' (1995: 104). Equity considerations, they recommend, should be a more important part of the NHS monitoring process.

Funding arrangements

The final dimension on which health services can be characterized is in terms of funding arrangements. The British NHS is funded, as we have seen, primarily from general taxation, although an element of funding comes from the national insurance system and is, consequently, employment-related (around 16 per cent (Allsop 1995: 74)). Funding from general taxation provides an effective and equitable way of financing health care that offers universal entitlement based on medical need. It also allows the government, at least in theory, to control the level of health service spending, although within the NHS family practitioner services were not cash-limited until the end of the 1980s. The existence of clear powers to regulate expenditure is clearly one of the reasons why, viewed in international terms, UK expenditure on health services is comparatively low.

There are, however, also a number of disadvantages in funding health services from general taxation. Most important is the fact the health care has to compete with other areas of expenditure, and when there is pressure to control public expenditure—a situation that has existed throughout the history of the NHS, but has been particularly strong since the mid-1970s—the NHS is likely to suffer. One solution would be hypothecated taxation for health care, since there is evidence that increasing taxation for health care would be more acceptable than a general increase in taxation. However, hypothecated taxation has only been accepted by British governments in a few special cases, and there is evidence from other countries that even where it is introduced and commitments are made that the expenditure will be applied exclusively for the service in question, such promises are regularly broken. An alternative would be to increase social insurance payments and derive a far higher proportion of NHS funding from this method (they could cover the health costs of those in work, with the remainder covered by general taxation). Treated as a form of quasi-hypothecated taxation this would pose no major problems as long as the resources were used for the NHS, but the danger would be the development of two-tier arrangements since not everyone pays national insurance, with differential access and arrangements for the insured and uninsured.

A further disadvantage, sometimes mentioned, which can arise from funding from general taxation (or social insurance) is that it can mean that too little attention is paid to the cost of providing specific services. Although professionals may be aware of cash limits where they exist, they may have little idea of what their interventions cost. And since patients do not have to pay for most services, they do not have to think in terms of the cost of the service they are requesting. However, the level of cost-consciousness of professionals can be increased or constraints set on their spending by other means, and other mechanisms can be used to restrain unnecessary and inappropriate demand from patients (not always entirely successfully). The need for GP referral to a specialist is one such mechanism, as is the existence of waiting-lists. Paying doctors by salary or capitation also helps to keep costs down, since there is no direct financial incentive from recommending a medical intervention as there is under fee-for-service arrangements.[21] Indeed, the record suggests that services funded centrally are typically less expensive (even if those involved are not always as cost-conscious) than when they are funded through insurance. Consequently, notwithstanding the drawbacks, there appears to be little case on either of these grounds for major changes in the funding regime of the NHS.

Conclusion

The most important characteristic of the NHS is the universal entitlement grounded in citizenship, which the introduction of limited charging has so far done little to modify except in relation to dentistry. Nonetheless, access is far from perfect, not least because some services are not available or not readily available on the NHS. The existence of private medicine alongside the NHS has had some adverse consequences for the service, but has not, for a variety of reasons, reduced loyalty to state services in the way that it has with education. The development of a new managerialism in the service since 1983 has challenged the extent of medical dominance, but medical dominance has never been monolithic, not least because the profession itself has always been divided in various ways and it has largely been hospital consultants who have held especial sway and influence. Whether the new primary care commissioning will challenge the dominance of consultants will depend on the way the groups are structured, the extent of their powers, and how they are used. The concentration on curative rather than preventive medicine in the NHS is marked, and although health promotion and clinical prevention have expanded the more vital public health medicine has, regrettably, all too little place. It could only be expanded by a new commitment to allocating some NHS posts to public health work. There are, however, few grounds for a change in the mode of NHS funding, notwithstanding the financial pressures it faces, pressures which are discussed more fully in Chapter 6.

Chapter 5

Understanding Health Care Systems: Managing Sickness

THE health care system of a country is the set of institutional arrangements that have as their objective the treatment of sickness and the maintenance of health. The particular character of a health care system can be understood and explained in a number of different ways. In this chapter I want to look at some of these ways by considering three key questions about health care arrangements. First, why do health and sickness in human society need to be managed? Second, what factors shape the content of health care? And, third, what factors structure the main organizational features of a health care system? As we shall see, consideration of these three questions provides a way of examining a range of theoretical ideas about the character of health care systems. I conclude the chapter with a discussion of the forces influencing the introduction and development of the British National Health Service.

The need for management

We tend to take it for granted that some care and support will usually be provided for those who are sick, since we accept that sickness and disease are associated with pain and suffering and that these should be eased if at all possible. Certainly the relief of pain and suffering have often been important motivations for the familial and charitable care of the sick and dying, and we do not have to search hard for cultural beliefs about the importance of caring for those who are ill. Christianity, for example, stresses the importance of caring for the sick and vulnerable, and biblical narratives, especially those of the miracles performed by Jesus, often have the cure of sickness at their centre. Such narratives reinforce the ethic of altruism that biblical texts seek to propagate. In Britain as in other societies, therefore, where such religious beliefs still have some cultural force, they underpin institutional health care arrangements and the work of health practitioners.[1] Yet health care arrangements cannot be explained solely in such terms. Altruistic beliefs and altruism are important in understanding the response to sickness, but we also need to consider the problems sickness poses for society, whether the family, the local community, or the wider society, and why the maintenance of health is usually held to be important for the society as a whole.

Talcot Parsons (1951) has provided one of the most illuminating and influential analyses of sickness and health as problems for society—an analysis grounded in his structural functionalist approach to society. As Ute Gerhardt (1989) noted, Parsons offers two models of health and illness, and both contribute to the understanding of why health and illness need to be managed and of the way in which their boundaries are set. The first, the *capacity model*, is a formalization of the type of functional model of health and illness that we find in lay thinking in which health is often viewed as the capacity to cope with everyday activities (Blaxter 1990: ch. 2)—or, in more Parsonian language, it is the capacity to perform one's social roles satisfactorily.[2] In this model, illness is defined as states that undermine the performance of social roles—they are conditions that prevent us carrying out our daily routines properly—and it is the adequacy of social functioning that determines whether we judge mental or physical states as illnesses. Health and illness need to be managed because of the threat illness poses to society, since it stops individuals fulfilling their allocated tasks, which are essential to social stability and continuity. Societies and social groups have, therefore, necessarily to deal with illness. We may empathize with pain and suffering and genuinely want to care for the sick for their own sake, but as a social group we also need, if possible, to return sick individuals to health in order to restore the smooth functioning of the group. Indeed, sickness poses a dual threat, since it not only incapacitates the sick but also uses up the time and energies of those who provide care.[3]

Parsons's capacity model of health and illness has a number of merits. First, it asserts the intimate relation between individual functioning, the functioning of society, and definitions of ill-health, and in that respect makes it very clear why health and illness can create problems for society and may require social regulation, not just at the level of the family but at the level of the wider society. The social control of sick individuals is necessary for the smooth functioning of society and though we may care for the sick we also control them. Indeed, in advanced industrial societies, sickness legitimates some of the strictest of social regulations. Sickness, because it can mean the non-performance of social roles, is a potential threat to the social system, and so needs to be regulated and legitimated (most visible in sickness certification for those in paid work) and efforts made to reintegrate the individual back into society.

Second, the incapacity model highlights the importance of social norms—expectations and standards of social behaviour—in definitions of health and illness. What is considered illness or incapacity in one group will not necessarily be the same in another. This is the point about variations in boundaries and thresholds of illness over time and between societies made on an empirical basis in Chapter 1. Here the significance is not just the variation in standards but the indication that such variation is linked to social regulation, to the maintenance of social order, and to the smooth functioning of society. Third, the incapacity model fits with a further important feature of lay understandings of illness. This is the assumption that a person is *unable* to perform their usual tasks: that their illness is something that happens to them and is not a matter of will, at least once they are ill. However much a person may be blamed for becoming ill, agency is not assumed. Passivity is embedded in the very terminology of illness as, most obviously, in the term 'patient'.

Fourth and most importantly, it allows us to see that the significance of illness is likely to vary according to the social role of the sick person—the threat that the sickness of a given individual poses to a group depends on their place in that group and the roles they perform both present and future. It is noteworthy in this context that problems with the supply of recruits for the military has frequently been an important impetus for action about the population's health. In contrast, in terms of task performance sickness in the elderly may be less threatening than in, say, a breadwinner, though their care may pose significant problems. However, in a situation where the labour of breadwinners can easily be replaced because of a ready supply of labour, their sickness will be less threatening to the wider society than to their own family. Children are an interesting category here: their incapacity may be of little immediate importance in terms of task performance, but they represent an investment in the future, and their illness may be seen as a threat to the society's future supply of healthy adults as well as creating extra work for those who have to care for them.[4]

Parsons's second model of illness, *illness as deviance*, is linked to one of his key analytic contributions—his concept of the sick role. Parsons asserts that whilst illness usually involves non-performance of customary social roles it is itself also a social role. Illness is consequently not only a set of material, bodily processes which constitute the disease, it is also, once recognized, itself a social role governed by its own set of expectations. The central expectation is, according to Parsons, that by virtue of their illness, and depending on its severity, individuals will, to a greater or lesser extent, be exempt from their usual social obligations. However, at the same time they will be expected, he argues, to seek medical help if appropriate in an effort to get well, and to do what is required of them to achieve this end. Parsons's analysis therefore assumes the existence of a medical profession whose job it is to help the sick recover from their illness. But this assumption is not crucial to the argument at this point. What is important is the idea that illness is associated with exemption from normal social obligations, since it this that underpins his deviance model of illness.

In Parsons's deviance model it is the exemption from major, everyday social obligations which allows the claim that illness can be viewed as a form of deviance—that is, a form of rule-breaking. This is because, whilst we tend to associate illness with pain and suffering and consequently see it as a negative state (indeed, as we have seen, its undesirability is inherent in the concept itself), analysing it in terms of social obligations shows us the positive features of being ill. And once we have taken this step, it forces us to recognize that individuals may be motivated to illness in order to achieve exemption from social obligations or any other gains associated with being ill. We may wish, consciously or unconsciously, to be ill in order to avoid certain responsibilities, to get attention, to put ourselves in a situation of dependence, or to require others to look after us or to treat us better. And if this is the case then we can also view illness as motivated action and the sick person as breaking social rules in failing to fulfil their social obligations.

Moreover, according to Parsons, illness as a form of deviance has certain rather important characteristics. On the one hand, it puts the individuals into a situation of dependence. Illness, he suggests, is 'predominantly a withdrawal into a dependent relation, it is asking to be "taken care of"' (1951: 285). On the other hand, it usually isolates the individual and exposes them to strong mechanisms of social control:

> the sick role involves a *relative* legitimacy, that is so long as there is an implied 'agreement' to 'pay the price' in accepting certain disabilities and the obligation to get well. It may not be immediately obvious how subtly this serves to isolate the deviant. The criminal, being extruded from the company of 'decent' citizens, can only by coercion be prevented from joining up with his fellow criminals . . . The conditional legitimation of the sick person's status on the other hand, places him in a special relation to people who are not sick, to the members of his family and to the various people in the health services, particularly physicians. This control is part of the price he pays for his partial legitimation, and it is clear that the basic structure resulting is that of the dependence of each sick person on a group of non-sick persons rather than of sick persons on each other. (Parsons 1951: 312)

Parsons's deviance model, even more than the incapacity model, emphasizes therefore the dimension of social control and regulation by pointing to the motivational elements involved in illness. To the extent that individuals are agents in their own illness, then regulation needs to be tighter and illness is potentially a greater threat. The deviance model also helps us to understand the ongoing tensions in the assumptions we make about sick individuals: between viewing them as victims of misfortune, with the denial of agency of the incapacity model, and as somehow to blame for their situation as in the deviance model.

Nonetheless, Parsons's claim that all illness can be viewed as a form of deviance raises problems. In particular, even accepting the importance of unconscious motivation (Parsons's analysis drew heavily on Freud), it is far from clear that all illness involves sufficient motivational components for us to view it as a form of deviance, despite the fact that, once an individual is ill, when the sick role is occupied, motivational components do inevitably enter the picture.

Parsons's analysis of illness in terms both of incapacity and of deviance provides us therefore with some very important clues as to why illness and health need to be regulated, and starts to indicate the conditions under which a society may become more or less involved in their regulation, including playing a part in the provision of health care—ideas that have been taken up by other writers offering analyses of health care systems. For example, a number of Marxist writers in the 1970s used a similar functionalist framework in seeking to understand the management of illness; however, instead of emphasizing the functional value of its management to society as a whole, they stressed the functions of health care to the capitalist economy. One function mentioned by some Marxists is its role in the maintenance of human capital—that is, the labour necessary for production (Rodberg and Stevenson 1977: 112). Here health care is viewed as a form of investment in the labour of individuals which can bring economic returns, though whether it does or not will depend on the cost of the health care, its efficacy, and the value of the workers in question (how skilled they are, etc). Where jobs are mostly unskilled and there is a ready supply of unskilled labour, and where health care is relatively ineffective, then there will be little return from health care spending.[5]

A rather different argument, again drawing on the tradition of Marxism and political economy (and also on Parsonian foundations), can be used to suggest that the boundaries of health are set in relation to the needs of the labour market. A number of writers have, for instance, argued that the size of the in-patient mental hospital population can be linked to the health of the economy and the demand for labour (Brenner 1973; Warner 1994). When the economy is thriving and there is a considerable demand for labour, then the boundaries of acceptable psychological health are set more broadly and the psychiatric in-patient population declines. When the economy is less buoyant or in recession, then the demand for labour slackens and more people are likely to end up as psychiatric in-patients. The same analysis can be applied to other forms of ill-health, particularly where it is chronic (see e.g. Bartley 1993; Rowlingson and Berthoud 1996).

A further argument frequently developed in the Marxist literature is that health care plays an important ideological role, especially in legitimating capitalism by making people believe the system is capable of meeting their needs. Vicente Navarro, whose ideas about the causes of illness were outlined in Chapter 2, is one of those who developed this argument, contending that health care helps to legitimate capitalism by transforming the problems it generates into individual problems (the echoes of Parsons's argument about the way in which illness is an individualizing form of deviance are strong). For example:

> the social utility of medicine is measured primarily in the arena of systemic legitimation. Medicine is indeed socially useful, to the degree that the majority of people believe and accept the proposition that what are actually politically-caused conditions can be individually solved by medical intervention. And, from the point of view of the capitalist system, this is the actual utility of medicine; it contributes to the legitimation of capitalism. It is because of this legitimation function that the medical profession is serving the interests of the capitalist system and of the capitalist class. (Navarro 1977: 69)

A rather different theoretical approach is provided by Michel Foucault, who talks not of the capitalist state, conceived as a coherent, calculating subject, but in terms of 'governmentality'. Foucault argues that from the beginning of the eighteenth century a science of government directed towards the economy (viewed at the level of the state) developed—a science whose object was the processes relating to the population and its welfare: improvements in its conditions, its health, wealth, and longevity. He terms this development 'governmentality', one of whose meanings is:

> The ensemble formed by the institutions, procedures, analyses and reflections, the calculations and tactics that allow the exercise of this very specific albeit complex form of power, which has as its target population, as its principal form of knowledge political economy, and as its essential technical means apparatuses of security. (Foucault 1991: 102)

Governmentality, of which attention to the health of the population is an integral component, pervades modern societies, Foucault contends, and depends on the institutionalization of expertise in which the professions, including the health care professions, play a crucial part. However, conceived in this way, governmentality might be expected to be associated far more with public health medicine, with its concern for populations and societal changes, than with clinical medicine, or the individually oriented health promotion and clinical prevention that has largely replaced it. The dominance of individually oriented preventive work is due, I suggested in the last chapter, to a number of factors, including the power of the medical profession. Such considerations direct us therefore towards examination of the role of health care professionals, and to the explanation of the characteristics of health care systems which I discuss in the next two sections. Let us turn therefore to my second question: what factors structure the content of health care?

Professionalizing strategies and the content of health care

In thinking theoretically about the content of health care within a particular society, we need to start by considering the providers of health care and then look at the factors that shape the character of their work, since the two are interrelated.

The informal, unpaid care provided within families or close social networks has always been a major component of health care provision. Family members, often women, routinely provide care for the sick as well as contributing to the maintenance of their own and their families' health through their domestic labour, by cooking meals, cleaning homes, clothes, and bodies, and giving advice and guidance (Stacey 1988). However, typically societies also allocate special powers and responsibilities to some individuals to act as advisers and healers in the care and treatment of sickness, and these official healers play a key role in shaping the content of specialized health care. For example, shamans who are held to have magical powers have been significant figures in some societies in relation to the sick. In Western societies a parallel role has often been played by those within the church who have drawn on a range of religious and magical beliefs in their treatment (see MacDonald 1981). And once beliefs in the supernatural begin to disappear this role is carried out by a range of healers, often very numerous. For example, estimates of the numbers of healers practising in Norwich (then the second largest city in the country) in the sixteenth century suggest that there was one healer for every 220 to 250 persons (Pelling and Webster 1979). Healing was for the most part a trade and healers plied their potions, medicines, and advice in the market place.

In Britain from the sixteenth century onwards, and even before, we can see two processes occurring. First, there was an increasing regulation and professionalization of healers and healing, with a growing differentiation between official, licensed healers and those whose activities were not licensed. It was in this context that the medical profession developed, a grouping of those who increasingly managed to secure recognition as official healers. And second, there was an increasing division of labour within healing. In the sixteenth-century marketplace there was already some division of labour amongst healers. On the one hand, there were divisions between the physicians, barber-surgeons, and apothecaries, groups whose early professionalizing endeavours were mentioned in the previous chapter, and who included licensed as well as unlicensed healers. On the other hand, there were women specializing in childbirth, the nascent profession of midwifery on the fringe of official medicine (Pelling and Webster 1979), as well as others such as itinerant herbalists and bone-setters. Handywomen and domestic servants were also paid to help with the care of the sick, and those employed to help with domestic duties were the group from whom the nursing profession emerged—a development given impetus by the establishment of voluntary hospitals in the first half of the eighteenth century.

Theoretically the professionalization of healing, which was crucial to the emerging character of health care, can be understood in a number of different ways. Early discussions of the professions tended to see them as occupational groups with certain distinctive characteristics or traits, such as adherence to a professional code of conduct, the provision of training, skills based on theoretical knowledge, and altruism (Johnson 1972: 23). Later discussions have tended to emphasize that professionalization is a process, and to analyse the strategies occupational groups use to professionalize themselves, seeing the particular patterning of the powers and distribution of health care providers as the outcome of struggles between professional groups, in which they have sought support from the public and the state in legitimating and sustaining their activities. Analyses informed by Weberian ideas, which see professionalization as part of the rationalization and bureaucratization of society, have been highly influential. For Eliot Freidson (1970; 1994) the major objective of a profession such as medicine is to achieve autonomy—that is, freedom from the control of outsiders. This autonomy is to be found in the power to regulate the education and training of its members, including the content of the curriculum, the power to determine who is a member of the profession, and the power to regulate members' conduct and to hold disciplinary hearings. Autonomy, whose extent and nature varies over time, is granted by the state and has to be secured. Freidson refers to a number of tactics which helped to give the medical profession autonomy: these included the ability to secure 'good results' in its work—i.e. some success in its treatments; 'a sound foundation of knowledge' in which the deployment of science played a crucial part; and the ability to secure the backing of the elite in society (1970: 21). In this process it was support and persuasion and the perception of skills and expertise, the latter strongly allied to claims about the scientific character of medical work, that counted even more than actual achievements. Consequently the developing character of medical work, in particular its focus on the sick and its use of science, are intimately linked to medicine's efforts to secure professional power.

Freidson notes that medical power has a second important source: the authority that derives from office: that is, from the fact that doctors have a formal position within the health services which gives them certain legal powers exclusive to that office, powers that do not depend directly on their expertise, although presumptions of expertise are crucial to the allocation of such powers (the acquisition of office also gives rise to presumptions of expertise). In the case of medicine, the powers of office include the power to admit patients to hospital, to issue medical certificates, to sign death certificates, and to issue prescriptions for certain drugs. These formal powers are a very important foundation of doctors' power over patients and may be used to help to ensure patient compliance.

Drawing on the Weberian tradition and emphasizing the importance of social stratification, Larson developed such ideas further, offering a dynamic model of the 'professional project' of an occupational group, and arguing that a group tries to use its knowledge and expertise in order to enhance its income and standing and to secure a monopoly position within the labour market:

> Professionalization is thus an attempt to translate one order of scarce resources—special knowledge and skills—into another—social and economic reward. To maintain scarcity implies a tendency to monopoly: monopoly of expertise in the market, monopoly of status in a system of stratification. (Larson 1977: p. xvii)

What is suggested here is an active imperialism in which the profession seeks to pursue its own economic and social interests by exploiting its knowledge and skills, so placing expertise and claims to expertise centre stage. Other writers have analysed professionalizing strategies in terms of the processes of social closure adopted by an occupational group. For Parkin (1979), modes of occupational closure are different means of mobilizing power so that a group can stake claims to resources and opportunities. The group seeks to maintain or strengthen its dominance by defining clear boundaries between itself and other groups which it aims to put or keep in a subordinate situation, setting clear boundaries around those who belong to the group and excluding others. For example, in the case of medicine, those who fall outside its boundaries may be excluded and denigrated by being defined as 'charlatans' or 'quacks'. Or they may be portrayed as having a legitimate but clearly differentiated and subordinate place in the healing process. Not surprisingly, boundaries tend to be continually contested and the struggle between occupational groups is ongoing.

Witz (1992), drawing on the work of Freidson (1970), Parkin (1979), and Murphy (1984), distinguishes four types of professionalizing strategy: the exclusionary and demarcationary strategies employed by the dominant occupational group which involve the downward exercise of power, and the inclusionary and dual closure strategies employed by the subordinate group which exert a countervailing upwards exercise of power by those subject to exclusionary and demarcationary strategies. Inclusionary strategies involve attempts to secure inclusion in activities from which the group is excluded, and dual closure strategies involve attempts to consolidate one's own position when subject to demarcationary strategies by trying both to usurp the dominant group and to exclude subordinate groups. Witz provides a largely historical analysis of the strategies of four professional groups: doctors, midwives, nurses, and radiographers. What is important is not, however, fitting the strategies used by particular occupational groups into the categories, but awareness and sensitivity to the professionalizing strategies used by specific occupational groups.

Witz further argues that gender plays an important part in professionalizing strategies, and that the concept of profession is itself gendered. This is because its meaning has been constructed around the work and activities of specific male occupational groups with a distinctive class position: 'it takes what are in fact the successful professional projects of class-privileged male actors at a particular point in history and in particular societies to be the paradigmatic case of profession' (Witz 1992: 39). Historically, part of what it meant to be a professional was to be a 'gentleman': a man with a particular standing in the world. It also meant a level of commitment to one's work that was only possible for those who could rely on the domestic labour of others (usually wives or servants) to sustain their bodily needs, and where success was facilitated by a wife's administrative and secretarial (and at times social) support (Finch 1983). These connotations of the term 'profession' still remain, albeit in an attenuated form.

Medicine's use of science and technology, which I discussed in the previous chapter, provides an illustration of the use of exclusionary and demarcationary strategies as part of its professional project. It also shows the way in which professionalizing strategies are bound up with and shape the content of medical work. The process of professionalization not only structures the particular constellation of health practitioners that emerges at a particular moment of time, it also helps to structure the content of health care. In the sixteenth and seventeenth centuries physicians' claims to expertise were based on their classical learning. Subsequently doctors have generally used the natural sciences to provide the basis for their claims to expertise and the foundation of their exclusionary and demarcationary strategies against other groups of healers. And in so doing they have encouraged the clinical focus of medicine and other health care work, the curative bias of health services, as well as the enthusiasm for high technology procedures, and the prestige and dominance of hospital-based work. This means not just a concentration on certain types of work—curing sick individuals where possible through the use of advanced science—but also some selectivity in which patients receive medical care. As Sir Keith Joseph commented when Minister of Health, 'Doctors can be remarkably selective in choosing the ills they regard worthy of treatment' (quoted in Klein 1989: 81). However, medicine's use of science is not to be viewed here as something external to the profession which they appropriate, but as a knowledge that they themselves construct and develop, whose status they help to determine, and which they deploy in their claims-making activities as part of their professional project. By virtue of their education and training doctors could claim special expertise in the natural sciences and scientific knowledge of the workings of the body, even though the character of clinical practice, with its focus on the individual, ensured that agreed scientific principles were often compromised. The result has been the dominance of bio-medicine within current health care arrangements.

The introduction of Project 2000 nurse training in the late 1980s and 1990s provides a further example of professionalizing strategies and the way in which they shape the work of health care practitioners. P2000 offered a new model of basic nurse training which had two important characteristics in relation to nursing knowledge and expertise. First, the academic component was far stronger than in the earlier training, the aim being to treat nurses as students for three years rather than as on-the-job apprentices who contributed to the work of the ward. Second, P2000 training attempted to articulate and develop a somewhat more distinctive knowledge base for the profession, stressing nurses' specialist knowledge of health as opposed to illness (with which medicine is usually associated) and adopting a bio-psycho-social approach (in contrast to medicine's common focus on the biological). It is not yet clear how successful this strategy has been, or how extensive its impact on the work of nurses has been, but nursing's professionalizing strategies have frequently not been very successful, not least because of the power of the historically male medical profession to keep female nursing as the handmaiden of medicine (see Witz 1992: ch. 5; Davies 1995). Moreover, nurses' terms and conditions of work have been tightly controlled by their employers (unlike doctors, they do not have a strong 'independent practitioner' model), which has further curtailed their power.

Theoretically such analyses of the work of clinicians and the content of health care are largely informed by Weberian theorizing about the professions, and such theorizing has not escaped criticism. From a Marxist perspective, Navarro in *Medicine under Capitalism* (1976) argued that this type of theorizing attributed too much power to the professions, including too much power in the shaping of the content of health care. Doctors, he contended, play a part as professionals in the health care system but they are not the owners and controllers of the system, merely the administrators. It is capitalism and the capitalist state that shape the health care system, not the activity of the professions, which inevitably play a subordinate role (though in later discussions (see Navarro 1978) he indicated that they did play some part in shaping health services). Navarro's analysis in *Medicine under Capitalism* differs, therefore from Freidson's in respect to the autonomy of the medical profession (see also McKinlay 1977). For Freidson, autonomy has to be granted by the state, but even where the state comes to control the terms and conditions of work (as in state health care), the profession still retains clinical autonomy. For Navarro, power is located in the capitalist state not the medical profession. However, it is important to note in this context the increasing commercialization of medicine and health care in both the United States (Starr 1982; Salmon 1985) and Britain. Business corporations increasingly recognize that many aspects of health care—health insurance, drugs, bio-technology, medical equipment, building and running hospitals—can offer enormous commercial opportunities, and some are playing a growing part in providing, and shaping, health care.

Foucault's analysis of governmentality (1991) has also been used to call into question some elements of Freidson's and others' theorizing. For instance, Johnson has argued that the dualism Freidson assumes between profession and state is unsatisfactory. Rather, the professions need to be viewed as part of the process of governmentality, and as such as part of the state not distinct from it: 'the modern professions emerged as part of that apparatus that constitutes the state' (Johnson 1995: 12). Such an argument has echoes of Navarro's analysis, since it appears to view the professions as agents of state activity. However, they have very different conceptions of the state. For Navarro, the state is 'a configuration of public institutions and their relationship' which is not only an explicitly capitalist state with a clearly defined set of interests (its 'primary role is the reproduction of an economic system based on private ownership of the means of production' (Navarro 1976: 116)), but is also attributed a degree of agency. For Foucault, as we have seen, the state is defined rather broadly as the ensemble of institutions, procedures, calculations, and tactics that allow the exercise of governmentality. He therefore includes the professions and professional expertise as components of the state rather than as separate from it. Moreover, his is not a distinctively capitalist state with distinctively capitalist interests, nor is it attributed the same degree of agency—it is not a coherent, calculating subject.

Of course, Foucault's analysis of governmentality and the state is not without its problems. The monolithic version of the state wedded to capitalist interests in Marxist accounts may have its flaws, and Foucault's conception, which recognises disunity, conflicting interests, and lack of common purpose, appears to fit empirical reality rather better. But the danger is that the state is defined too broadly with little in the way of potential empirical precision. Moreover, there is not only too little sense of agency and interests but also too little concern for the relations between components of the state.[6] Macdonald (1995: 24–7) argues that Foucault's conception of governmentality is at a level of abstraction that makes it of little value to those interested in empirical analyses of the professions. This view is not, however, shared by Johnson, who suggests that Foucault's analysis of governmentality generates processual models in which, for instance, the boundaries between the technical (clinical) and the political are explored. Yet much of what Johnson suggests is consistent with, and indeed contained within, sociological accounts such of as those of Freidson and Larson.

Two important points emerge from these theoretical debates. First, that it is essential to retain a dynamic, processual view of professional activities. Second, that in order to understand the activities of the health professions and the structuring of clinical work we need to pay attention to the power of a range of different actors. On one hand, we need to examine the professional struggle between the occupational groups involved in healing: doctors, nurses, midwives, pharmacists, and so forth. On the other, we need to examine the struggles between professional groups and other sources of power, notably the state and commercial companies.

In order to provide a dynamic framework for analysing the professions, Donald Light (1995) uses the notion of 'countervailing powers', a framework which recognizes that the extent of the power of the different health professions varies over time and that other forces, including the state, play an important role in their development. In his simplest model he analyses a profession's power on two axes: one ranging from professional dominance at one end to state dominance at the other, the second ranging from independent employment at one end and state employment at the other. He notes, however, that such a model needs to be broadened to include other actors, such as the media.

The pharmaceutical industry is one such countervailing power. The industry is now dominated by large-scale companies with global markets which operate on a highly commercial basis; some are amongst the largest companies in the world and several are multinationals (Abraham 1995). Their influence and power *vis-à-vis* the medical profession is enormous, and their decisions as to where potential profits are to be made in developing new drugs (or replicating existing ones—many drugs fall into the 'me too' category) help to shape health care. However, the relationship between medicine and the pharmaceutical industry is highly symbiotic. On the one hand, drugs provide key weapons in the therapeutic armoury of medical practitioners who have secured monopoly powers to prescribe some drugs, which as I have noted is an important source of their professional power (in relation both to expertise and to office). Consequently, pharmaceutical companies play a key role in sustaining the power and legitimacy of the medical profession. On the other hand, the pharmaceutical industry depends on the support of doctors as well as potential patients in its search for markets for its products. Not surprisingly, therefore, the issue of the regulation of the drugs industry is of considerable importance and, given the global character of the industry, far from easy. In Britain the Committee on the Safety of Medicines, set up in 1963 following the thalidomide tragedies, makes recommendations on licensing new products. However, these requirements are not very extensive (see Chapter 6). Yet once licensed few drugs have had their licence suspended (the arthritis drug Opren is one example). There is also the problem of regulatory capture (Abraham 1995: 22–4) which is compounded in the case of the drugs industry by its importance in maintaining medical power.

Patients are another group mentioned by Light who play a role in shaping health care, sometimes supporting and sometimes counterbalancing the powers of clinicians. In the first place, the bias towards curative medicine is often encouraged and sustained by the sick and their families. The sick, and those who feel threatened by the risk of sickness, can articulate a strong voice, which is usually directed towards putting resources into treating those who are ill, and only occasionally towards prevention—for instance, when illness is seen as a high risk (the panics surrounding AIDS are a recent example, but so too were the nineteenth-century concerns of the middle and upper classes at the threats of infectious illnesses such as cholera, which were no respecters of persons).[7]

Second, patients and patient groups play a role in shaping specific aspects of the content of health care and in pressing the case for particular types of provision. Within the NHS users are formally given only a limited advisory role as members of Community Health Councils, which were first introduced in the 1974 reorganization and have arguably seen their powers diminish as a result of the 1990 reorganization. However, users exert their power in other ways. Of particular interest has been the growth of organized user groups, often composed of patients and former patients and/or their families. These usually focus on a particular illness which they consider is not being adequately provided for, in terms either of the levels of funding or of the types of treatment that are offered, or in the ways that the condition is being understood. Some groups concentrate on providing, information, advice, and support. Others take an active political role, sometimes highly critical of the medical profession. Examples of politically active groups in Britain include the Disability Alliance, MIND (the National Association for Mental Health), SANE (schizophrenia, a national emergency, though now with a broader brief), Alcohol Concern, the National Childbirth Trust, the two ME (myalgic encephalitis) groups—Action for ME and ME Action (Cooper 1998)—the National Abortion Campaign (NAC),

Body Positive (an HIV/AIDS campaigning group), and various cancer groups including the UK Breast Cancer Coalition. To this list could be added the activities of the women's health movement, which established a number of women's health clinics and well women clinics—a model then copied more widely by GP practices, initially for women and then for men.[8] Theoretically we can understand the work of such groups in a number of different ways. For instance, they can be analysed in terms of resistance to medical power or by drawing on the literature of pressure groups and the newer work on new social movements.

The subjective experience of illness is frequently a key issue for patients. Whereas the earlier bedside medicine held patients' experiences to be a vital source of information in understanding illness and disease, biomedicine with its mechanistic approach has tended to focus on what can be observed and measured, whether on the surface of the body or inside. In consequence, subjective experience has been given less attention. Yet critics have argued that this lack of attention to subjective experience carries a double disadvantage. First, insofar as it affects the relationship between patient and practitioner it means that the patient may be less willing or less able to convey information which may be crucial to accurate diagnosis. Second, since psychological states may be very important to the therapeutic process, if the patient's experiences are ignored the chances of successful treatment are reduced. A number of classic studies have argued the case for greater attention to patients' experiences. For example, the psychiatrist R. D. Laing, in his influential study of schizophrenia, *The Divided Self* (1960), provided a phenomenological account of the experience of schizophrenia and went on to berate psychiatrists for the lack of attention to experience (1967). More recently the anthropologist Arthur Kleinman has called for far greater attention to the 'narratives of illness' provided by patients (1988), particularly those with chronic illness, arguing for their importance to the therapeutic process.

The organization of health care systems

The theoretical ideas presented in the first two sections of this chapter are very relevant to the third and final question concerning the forces that structure the organization of a particular health care system. In the first section I explored theoretical ideas that offered rationales for the development of health care arrangements in a society; and in the second I examined ideas about the professionalizing projects of health practitioners which have an impact on the character of a given health care system, especially the content of health care.

We need now to look at ways of understanding the organization of health systems.

Theoretically, in order to understand the organizational development of a health care system we need to locate that system within the welfare arrangements of the society, which Esping-Andersen (1990) calls its welfare regime. It is these welfare regimes that underpin and help to explain the particular character of the health system. Esping-Andersen distinguishes three main types of welfare regime within present-day European societies: the liberal, the corporatist, and the social democratic. These ideal types are differentiated partly according to the character of the regime and the basis of entitlement to welfare—citizenship, employment status, and financial need, the typology I introduced in describing the British health system in the previous chapter—and partly according to the political philosophies underpinning them which add an important explanatory component. In analysing his three regimes Esping-Andersen uses the concept of de-commodification. Commodification refers to the situation where the welfare of individuals depends on the market; de-commodification to the process where welfare becomes a matter of right and survival does not depend on participation in the market (an analysis that has clear Marxist overtones).

The first regime Esping-Andersen outlines is the liberal welfare regime grounded in *laissez-faire* principles that we associate with Victorian Britain:

> Benefits cater mainly to a clientele of low-income, usually working-class, state dependents. In this model, the progress of social reform has been severely circumscribed by traditional, liberal work-ethic norms: it is one where the limits of welfare equal the marginal propensity to opt for welfare instead of work. Entitlement rules are therefore strict and often associated with stigma; benefits are typically modest. In turn, the state encourages the market, either passively—by guaranteeing only a minimum—or actively—by subsidizing private welfare schemes. (Esping-Andersen 1990: 26–7)

Such a regime minimizes de-commodification effects and 'erects an order of stratification that is a blend of relative equality of poverty among state-welfare recipients, market-differentiated welfare among the majorities, and a class-political dualism between the two' (p. 27)). Esping-Andersen identifies the US, Canada, and Australia as the archetypes of this model but also suggested, writing in 1990, that Britain, whose nineteenth-century Poor Law provision was an instance of a liberal welfare regime, was falling back into this category (the actual welfare regime of any particular country is likely to combine elements from more than one ideal type).

When applied to health care the liberal welfare regime means a system of health care dependent on the financial ability to take out the necessary insurance (which may be part of an employment package and whose scope will vary).

This private, market-based health care is usually backed up by a residual publicly financed system of health care for those not covered by insurance and for types of care that are excluded (usually long-term care) with entitlement based on financial need.[9] This is essentially the system in the United States where 39 million people were not covered by private insurance in 1992 (some 71.4 per cent of those under 65) and another 40 million were under-insured especially in relation to serious illness (Skocpol 1996: 16). Such people are dependent for health care either on Medicare, a scheme for the elderly, or Medicaid, a scheme for the poor, both state-funded.

The second type of European welfare state regime Esping-Andersen delineates is the corporatist. In these welfare states the obsession with market efficiency and commodification is not so predominant. Instead:

> What predominated was the preservation of status differentials; rights, therefore, were attached to class and status. This corporatism was subsumed under a state edifice perfectly ready to displace the market as a provider of welfare. (Esping-Andersen 1990: 27)

Such regimes tend to be conservative and shaped by the church, often the Catholic Church. Consequently, they are usually committed to traditional models of the family; they tend to exclude non-working wives from social insurance, and make little provision in the way of child care. Examples of such regimes include Austria, France, Germany, and Italy.

Applied to health care this type of welfare regime means that entitlement to care is based on employment status and involves compulsory, state, employee-based health insurance schemes, introduced as a means of ensuring that all employees have some income when they are sick as well as access to medical care. Funding usually involves some combination of payment by the individual, the employer, and the state, and services often remain in private hands. The national insurance scheme that existed in Britain between 1911 and the establishment of the NHS followed this model, its major drawback typically being the exclusion of key groups: the elderly, the disabled, and frequently wives and children (in 1938 only 43 per cent of the British population were covered (Webster 1988: 11)).

Esping-Andersen's third type of welfare regime is the social democratic. In such regimes the principles of universalism operate:

> Rather than tolerate a dualism between state and market, between working class and middle class, the social democrats pursued a welfare state that would promote an equality of the highest standards, not an equality of minimal needs as was pursued elsewhere. This implied, first, that services and benefits be upgraded to levels commensurate with even the most discriminating tastes of the new middle classes; and, second, that equality be furnished by guaranteeing workers full participation in the quality of rights enjoyed by the better off. (Esping-Andersen 1990: 27)

All are incorporated into welfare arrangements although benefits may be graded according to earnings. Yet work is highly valued as are the capacities for individual independence; full employment is a key and essential commitment since employment is necessary for the realization of universal provision, and welfare arrangements usually allow women to enter the labour market. Consequently the market is still important, and the de-commodifiying elements of universal welfare are underpinned by continuing commodification. The main examples of this type of regime are to be found in Scandinavia. Esping-Anderson (1990: 53–4) also explicitly includes Beveridge's welfare state model, in which a universal health service was one component, in this category, but suggests that during the 1980s Britain fell back from the position it occupied in the period following the postwar welfare reforms. For instance, he describes Britain as a mixed case as far as pensions are concerned (1990: 87). However, in relation to its health care arrangements, Britain still falls clearly within his third type of regime, a situation that can in part be explained by the high level of public support for the NHS, and we can see very important elements of the social democratic welfare regime in the current Labour Government's welfare policies.

Universal schemes of state health care such as the NHS base entitlement on citizenship and make services available to all regardless of ability to pay, funding coming either from the insurance payments of those in employment (including contributions from employers) or from taxation (the main funding for the NHS). Such schemes usually develop out of compulsory employee insurance and may retain many of the elements of earlier arrangements (I noted in the last chapter the hybrid character of the NHS).

As is clear from the presentation of these three models, Esping-Andersen sees social class as central to any analysis of welfare regimes and regards the welfare state as part of the system of stratification. He argues that no single causal force can account for the emergence of the different types of welfare regime; rather, three factors are crucial. The first is: 'the nature of class mobilization (especially of the working class)' (Esping-Andersen 1990: 29). Here the focus is on social classes as agents of change, and the argument is that the balance of class power affects the way resources are distributed within the society. The second factor Esping-Andersen calls 'class-political coalition structures'—that is, the political alliances that can be created between social classes. The third is the 'historical legacy of regime institutionalization' (ibid. 1990: 29)—that is, the historical legacy of particular welfare arrangements which exist in a particular society at a given moment in time.

Esping-Andersen's emphasis on class mobilization and class coalitions has clear overtones of the Marxist focus on class struggle. Indeed, his analysis echoes some of the features of Navarro's (1978) analysis of the NHS in which he modified his earlier more functionalist approach and gave more explanatory importance to class struggle and the role of specific interest groups, including professional interests.[10] However, Esping-Andersen indicates that his own account differs from this type of Marxist position, partly because of his emphasis on class coalitions, but also because in his view welfare reforms themselves affect the balance of class power. Rather than simply helping to sustain capitalist power, they introduce contradictory elements that lessen workers' dependence on the market and potentially increase their power.

The development of the National Health Service

Esping-Andersen is not alone in asserting the need to focus on a theoretically informed analysis of the specificities of particular historical circumstances to account for the development of welfare institutions including health services. In the case of the British NHS there can be little doubt of the importance of the wartime situation in facilitating the formulation and implementation of Beveridge's social democratic welfare state (albeit with some modifications and compromises) and of the NHS in particular. What is clear is that the Second World War changed class and political alliances and allegiances during the 1940s. Slow to respond to threats posed by Nazi Germany and reluctant to rearm, when war came Britain played a crucial role (along notably with the Soviet Union and the United States). As the contemporary term 'the people's war' suggests (Calder 1969), the war secured widespread popular support and was seen as both necessary and just by the majority of the population. Social cohesion and solidarity were undoubtedly enhanced by the threats of invasion, by the introduction of rationing, and by the establishment of Local Defence Volunteers (later the Home Guard). Whilst class distinctions did not disappear, boundaries were partially fractured by the sense of shared predicament and shared purpose that encouraged a desire for a different social order from the prewar era, in which unemployment, which had created such suffering amongst the working classes in the 1930s, would be eradicated (as it had been by the war itself), welfare provisions would be more adequate, and inequalities reduced. The 1942 Beveridge Report reflected and incorporated these concerns, setting out proposals for a welfare state, and attracted enormous interest within the country (over half a million copies of the report and summary report were sold (Calder 1969: 528)). That many of the proposals were largely implemented, often in a somewhat modified form, can be attributed to the electoral success of the Labour Party in 1945, an election in which support for the party came from across the social spectrum.

It was these social and political changes that underpinned the introduction of the NHS which came into existence on 5 July 1948, some two years after the National Health Service Act. The new service took over, as I have noted, many of the organizational features of the existing services, differing primarily in the introduction of entitlement on the basis of citizenship and, secondarily, in the nationalization of all the major hospitals. The latter was Aneurin Bevan's solution to the problem of hospital doctors' opposition to the taking of hospitals into municipal control, which had been envisaged in many of the earlier plans for a national health service.

The subsequent history of the NHS has equally been shaped by social, political and economic forces. Rudolf Klein in the second edition (1989) of his valuable analysis of the history and politics of the NHS divided the forty years of its existence into four basic periods: the period of consolidation from 1948 through to 1958, in which the focus was on administering the status quo; the period of technocratic change from 1959 through to the mid-1970s, characterized by the search for efficiency and rationality; the period of disillusionment from 1975 through to 1982; and what he calls the period of modernisation from 1983 onwards.[11]

During the early years of the NHS, when Labour was still in power, the focus was on ensuring that the new system operated reasonably smoothly, and the main anxieties were financial, anxieties that have to be set in the context of the relative austerity of the early postwar years (there was heavy indebtedness to the US under the Marshall plan). Concerns about the cost of the NHS arose almost immediately when Bevan's original estimate of £176 million for the cost of the first year of the service, 1948–9, quickly proved inadequate; by December 1948 he was predicting expenditure of £225 million for the year.[12] This higher level of expenditure was due, he suggested, to two factors: initial high levels of demand due to health problems that people had not been able to afford to tackle before, particularly in the areas of dental and ophthalmic care; and the higher cost of salaries than anticipated. Bevan's belief that the demand for health care might settle down after an initial period of high demand, since free access to health care would improve the population's health, was one he shared with Beveridge, who in his 1942 report argued that as the unmet health needs of the population were catered for demand would decline. This belief has proved mistaken not only because the scope of what medicine can offer has changed, but also because the interaction between levels of health, the availability of services, and demands for health care is more complex than either Beveridge or Bevan recognized—an issue discussed in the next chapter. However, the anxieties generated in this period were sufficient to lead the

Government as early as 1949 to pass legislation giving it powers to introduce prescription charges, though Bevan then fought a successful battle against their actual introduction; when in 1951 the Labour Government decided they must introduce some charges they opted for charges for dental and optical services.

Rudolf Klein notes that the Treasury's anxieties about costs in the early years of the NHS were somewhat unnecessary. The Guillebaud Committee set up to examine the cost of the NHS reported that much of the anxiety aroused on that subject had been exaggerated, and that 'the rising cost of the Service in real terms during the years 1948 to 1954 was less than people imagined' (quoted in Klein 1995: 31). Indeed, expenditure on the NHS had actually fallen as a proportion of the national income in 1950–1. Part of the problem was the competition the NHS faced in securing funds at a time when there was heavy expenditure on housing and defence, a situation that was not helped, once Bevan was transferred from Health to the Ministry of Labour, by the relatively low status of the Ministry of Health. When the Conservatives were returned to power, although they accepted the NHS, they saw it as a heritage from Labour and did not value it very highly. Between 1951 and 1958 there were six Ministers of Health, and in 1952 the one-shilling prescription charge to which Bevan had objected so strongly was introduced (with significant exemptions).

The period of technocratic change spanning the 1960s through to the early 1970s was, Klein argues, characterized by the search for rationality and efficiency through planning. Significantly, the economic context was no longer one of overall economic scarcity—this was the period of affluence, or at least that is how it was seen by contemporaries, in which economic improvements in comparison with the immediate postwar years lead to a sense of optimism, though the economy was probably not as strong as was thought at the time. However, for a variety of reasons—notably demographic changes, the rising cost of labour, and medical advances—the cost of the NHS was increasing, and this encouraged the belief that services should be planned more carefully.

The moves towards planning concentrated on the hospital sector. During the first decade of the NHS capital investment had been minimal, and in their 1959 election manifesto the Conservatives promised a programme of hospital-building; the same year the British Medical Association produced a report advocating a ten-year hospital plan, and making assessments as to the numbers of beds that would be needed per head of the population. In 1962 Enoch Powell, the Minister of Health, published the Ministry's own Hospital Plan setting out norms for the provision of hospital beds of different types, and envisaged the building of ninety new hospitals over the decade—a vision that was not then to be realized, though capital investment did begin to expand. One problem, Klein suggests, was that the long time period for building new hospitals (around ten years) meant that the immediate political gains from spending money on buildings rather than on current expenditure were small. Doctors, too, tended to be more concerned about current expenditure, which affected their pay, rather than capital expenditure. Significantly, too, there was no voice for users' interests within the NHS at this stage.

This period of innovation culminated in the 1974 reorganization of the NHS—a reorganization that seemed to offer a way of enabling more rational planning of services which the frustrations of the attempts to plan during the 1960s had highlighted. The objective was to achieve greater unity in the health services by moving away from the tri-partite structure which now seemed a major handicap to efficient organization and rational planning. Instead of three parallel strands—primary care services, hospital services, and local authority services—there were to be three levels: the region, the area, and the district, in a hierarchical arrangement, with the old executive councils transformed into family practitioner committees with direct links to the area health authorities.

The context of Klein's next period, the period of disillusionment from 1975 through to 1982, was the economic crisis that began during the Conservative Government in the early 1970s and had its origins in the sharp rise in oil prices. This led to what has been called the 'fiscal crisis of the state' (O'Connor 1973) and to major concerns to reduce public expenditure. The key NHS policy documents during this period involved plans to secure greater control over the allocation of resources, and were to a considerable extent an inheritance from the planning objectives of the earlier period. In 1976 the Government published a document entitled *Priorities for Health and Personal Social Services* (DHSS 1976), which looked at resource allocation across broad areas of NHS work. It argued the case for more resources to go to services for those with mental illness, physical or mental handicap, and services for the children and elderly—all areas which had fared badly in resource allocation up till then. The same year the report of the Resource Allocation Working Party (1976) was published which introduced formulas for the allocation of resources across the country in an effort to shift funding away from historic patterns to a more equitable basis. The period ended with the second major reorganization of the NHS in 1982, which eliminated the area health authorities on the grounds that the organizational structure of the NHS was too complex and bureaucratic.

Klein's final period of modernization spans the period of the Thatcher government and has arguably continued through into the new Labour administration, at least in respect of the modernizing objectives. The period of Conservative administrations was dominated by a neo-liberal agenda combining an ideological hostility towards the public sector, a belief that models derived from business should be applied to public-sector bodies, and a desire to cut public expenditure. The period was marked in the early years by the short, influential Griffiths Report (DHSS 1983), which introduced the idea of appointing managers to run every NHS body, and a new emphasis on efficiency and effectiveness to be measured by a range of performance indicators. It culminated during the era of Conservative administrations in the 1990 NHS and Community Care Act, which introduced the division between purchasers and providers in an effort to introduce an internal market into the NHS. Health service providers who constituted themselves as trusts were given more independence than the directly managed hospital services, and were expected to compete alongside private-sector providers for annual contracts to supply services. The purchasers included the new GP fundholding practices, which were allowed to purchase some hospital services (mainly elective surgery) on their patients' behalf.

With the electoral success of Labour in 1997 there have been a number of changes. The new Government's plans for the NHS, set out in a White Paper, *The New NHS* (Secretary of State for Health 1997), included a shift away from the competitive ethos within the NHS and a return to greater cooperation, the eradication of GP fundholding and its replacement with primary care group commissioning, as well as the introduction of three-year purchasing contracts. The proposals retained therefore some of the elements of the Conservative Government's reorganization, but also included new proposals, some of which are already being introduced. The new primary care groups are being set up, and the regions, an established feature of the NHS are being reorganized. Notable here is the decision to establish a single region for the whole of London to replace the earlier segmented pattern in which London was divided into four parts, each combined with an extensive hinterland, which made integrated, rational planning for London very difficult. The NHS has also been given further resources, though the extent to which the funds are new is debated.

Conclusion

The character of health systems, both the content of the health care that is provided and the organizational features of the system, depend on a range of forces. What is striking is that in Britain during the twentieth century the organizational arrangements have increasingly tended to be determined primarily at the level of government and to be shaped by a range of social, political, and economic forces, including the historic legacy of earlier arrangements for delivering health care. In contrast, the content of health care that is provided has largely been determined by health care professionals and, more recently, the pharmaceutical industry an other medical corporations, along with the intermittent intervention of groups of service users who may from time to time act as important pressure groups. Theoretically we can understand the shaping of both the content of health care and its organization by drawing on a range of ideas, including ideas about the social significance of sickness, about professionalization and the use of science as a foundation for claims to expertise and authority, about corporate power, and about the development and character of welfare regimes.

Chapter 6

Determining Resource Allocation Priorities

PROVIDING adequate health care in the face of rising demands and expectations has become the central issue for most health care systems, the National Health Service no less than any other. One solution is to spend more money on health care, a strategy that has some force in Britain since health care spending is proportionately lower than in many other advanced Western societies, though in part the lower spending is due to a relatively cost-effective system of health care. Nonetheless, whilst the overall level of resources going to the NHS is undoubtedly important and arguably should be increased, the issue of rising demands and expectations also needs to be examined and confronted.[1] Many would now argue that there is a need for some form of explicit rationing of health care, in the sense of setting specified limits on what can be provided, even if considerably more resources are directed towards health services. Not all demands for health care, they contend, can be met even where funding levels are high. Indeed, it is frequently argued that health care demands are potentially infinite. Consequently, faced with the inevitable mismatch between 'infinite demands, finite resources' (Klein 1995: 30), or as some might prefer to put it, demands that escalate more rapidly than resources, some form of rationing is inevitable. The task is to find a reasonable and equitable system of rationing.

Rationing of health care is not, of course, new. All systems of health care involve some form of rationing. Private, market-based health care systems allocate care on the basis of ability to pay, and this form of allocation rations health care in terms of the individual's financial resources. Some individuals may be excluded altogether because they cannot afford the health care available on the market, and some may only be able to purchase health care when illness is very severe. Moreover, where the cost is covered through an insurance scheme, the company's rules may exclude certain persons (e.g. those with certain pre-existing illnesses) or may provide only limited coverage for certain illnesses (e.g. those requiring long-term care). Consequently the form of rationing that operates where health care is purchased in the market does not meet criteria of equity, since ability to pay is more important than health need in determining who gets health care—indeed, need, if it is costly to meet, may be grounds for exclusion from access to health care altogether. Despite this, the possibility of purchasing at least some health care in the market tends to be accepted as an inevitable, taken-for-granted feature of society, and in Britain allows the more affluent to escape some of the financial constraints placed on the NHS.

Whilst the rationale of the NHS when it was set up was to achieve equity by allocating care on the basis of health need, in practice there was some implicit rationing since resources were not unlimited. A range of devices operated to restrict supply and control or suppress demand in the face of cash-limited hospital, but not primary care, budgets (the latter were not cash-limited until the end of the 1980s). One mechanism was rationing by delay, since patients often had to wait to see a doctor (particularly specialists), since their number was limited. Another mechanism was rationing by exclusion, since GPs as gatekeepers to specialist services could decide that a patient was not sufficiently ill to merit a specialist referral or that someone else's needs were greater, so helping to regulate the pressure on hospitals. Such rationing, often based on knowledge of the pressures facing specialists and the need to restrict demand, was rendered less visible to the majority of the public primarily because decisions on access were made by GPs and specialists under the guise of clinical judgement. What was supposedly an objective assessment of the medical need for specialist services could be confounded by knowledge of the availability of the service and the practitioner's own biases about treatment priorities—processes often favouring younger, higher-status patients. A further form of rationing in the NHS has been by dilution—that is by providing some treatment or service but not the most effective—for instance, medication when an operation is needed.[2] The main difference between the earlier situation and the present day is the increasing call from many health managers and policy makers for explicit rationing to deal with the problem of rising demand and the increased costs of health care, as well as a call for greater openness and public debate on rationing.

However, the language of rationing has two disadvantages when considering the problems of escalating demands and limited resources. First, it can conjure up rather negative images of scarcity, restriction, and central control which often derive from the wartime rationing of food and petrol—images of having to manage with limited amounts, of not being able to get what you want, and of having other people interfere with your life. Consequently some health managers and policy makers, including the present Government, try to avoid the term 'rationing', seeing it as politically disadvantageous because it puts the focus on finite resources and puts them on the defensive; others contend that clarity and blunt speaking are important and that it is essential to make the public aware that resources are not unlimited and hard choices need to be made. In this context it is significant that the White Paper, *The New NHS* (Secretary of State for Health 1997), focused almost entirely on organizational issues, largely relating to service delivery. The word 'rationing' is not used, though the need for the new primary care groups to make choices about the use of health resources is mentioned. In my view the bluntness of the language of rationing is actually one of its attractions, since it is important to recognize the centrality of allocational issues in any discussion of health care provision and to make the criteria as clear as possible, even though openness may create more opposition and political difficulty than implicit rationing. Moreover, whilst the language of rationing does have negative connotations it also has positive ones, many also deriving from wartime rationing, which can generate images of equitable allocation for the common good in the face of adversity.

Nonetheless, there is a rather different and more important argument against the language of rationing: that it formulates the difficulty facing health services in terms of a simple economic model of demand and supply in which the problem is the imbalance between demand on the one hand, and the available resources that limit what can be supplied on the other. This model clearly has some advantages in the way it poses the problem since it frames it in such a clear and simple way; I have used this framework so far in this discussion and will continue to do so from time to time. However, there are also major problems with operating exclusively within the framework of this narrow economic model when thinking about the allocation of health care. In particular the model tends to treat both demand and supply as givens and to focus on matching the one to the other, rather than looking at the origins and content of the demand for health care and how it is generated, and at the content of what is being supplied. The model also tends to treat demand as a matter of individual preference, making no distinction between 'needs' and 'wants'. Neither of these is a very precise concept, but their imprecision does not mean that the distinction is not useful or important. Using the economic framework the question becomes one of finding a solution to the imbalance, either by finding more resources to increase the supply of services or by deploying the resources more efficiently or cheaply (for instance, avoiding administrative waste or using less skilled labour to deliver some services), or by rationing the limited supply that is available by excluding certain individuals or categories of treatment (for instance, allowing kidney dialysis only for individuals under a particular age). The latter strategy necessarily requires some attention to which demands should be accepted and provided for, but it does not encourage us to look at how demands are shaped or at the forces that underpin the character of what is being supplied, which can be very helpful in thinking about priority-setting. Indeed, there is a tendency to assume that all clinical work, because it constitutes health care activity, is necessarily good and desirable. But this is to confound the positive evaluation of the objectives—health—with positive evaluation of the means—clinical work. We cannot and should not assume that the means are necessarily the best, or even the most appropriate. A key question has to be: 'Are we doing the right things?' (Muir Gray 1997). Consequently, whilst the economic model sets up the problem in a neat and simple way, it does not help us to think about the solutions very constructively because it does not direct us to thinking about the generation of the demand for health care or the content and worth of what is being supplied, which are central to dealing with the imbalance between supply and demand.

In my view the language of priority-setting is preferable to that of rationing because it makes it absolutely clear that the issues are not just about how much care can be provided but about precisely what care is to be provided and how necessary it is. However, since the phrase 'priority-setting' is used very widely in many different policy contexts, it is important to be very clear about the types of priority-setting under consideration. The priority-setting with which I am concerned here is a matter of how resources are allocated: it is about who gets what. But the level and type of resource allocation at issue can vary enormously, and the different types of priority-setting need to be clearly distinguished. The implicit NHS rationing mentioned earlier was rationing at the individual level: the selection of individuals for particular forms of treatment: should this particular individual get a kidney dialysis or not?[3] This is a very important issue, but it needs to be distinguished from priority-setting at the level of types of treatment: should we spend more on hip replacements than, say, on heart bypass operations? Both also need to be distinguished from priority-setting in terms of the broad areas of work, such as debates about whether to spend more on the hospital sector or on primary care, or to spend more on, say, services for the mentally ill and less on those with acute illnesses. This latter issue has received attention within the NHS, notably in the White Paper *Priorities for Health and Personal Social Services* (DHSS 1976), which argued the case for greater spending on the services for mental illness, mental and physical handicap, the elderly, and children, on the grounds that they had been starved of NHS resources.[4] However, there was considerable reluctance to increase spending on such services at the expense of the other sectors of medicine, and little shift in spending patterns occurred.

The issue of allocating resources between regions and localities, which is another type of priority-setting, has also received explicit attention in the NHS, most famously in the Report of the Resource Allocation Working Party (1976). The Report developed complex formulas for resource allocation that not only included measures such as population size and age distribution but also took account of mortality, fertility levels, and marital status. Whilst some progress was subsequently made towards RAWP targets, rather different formulas are now used for the geographical allocation of resources. Finally, there is priority-setting at the national level between different fields of welfare and between other areas of public expenditure, where the health services have to compete with education, social security, crime, and defence. The five types of priority-setting are set out in Table 6.1. In the discussion that follows I focus on types 4 and 5; treatment and individual priority-setting, since these are the areas where we have to look particularly carefully at the content of health care. As we shall see, these two types of priority-setting soon get intermingled, since comparison of different treatments quickly gets us into consideration of priority-setting at the individual level. Indeed, I shall argue that in many cases priority-setting has to operate at the level of individuals and their specific problems rather than through general rankings of types of treatment.

However, whilst I shall deploy the language of priority-setting because it indicates very clearly the need for evaluation and choices, it is important to note that this language still tends to have rather little to say about the ways in which the demands for health care and the content of health care are shaped. What is needed is a more complex, more sociological analysis that recognizes that demand and supply should not be treated as givens but as the outcome of social processes, which makes a distinction between health problems and the demand for health care, and which analyses critically the content and direction of medical work. Spending on some types of health care, even if demanded, may not be appropriate whether the money is coming from government or the private purse.

In the previous chapter I outlined some of the theoretical ideas about the ways we can seek to understand the shaping of the content of health care through notions such as professionalization and through broader models such as Light's (1995) idea of countervailing powers. In this chapter I focus on four broad areas: on the ways in which the demand and supply of health care are

Table 6.1 Types of resource allocation priority-setting

1. Public expenditure priority-setting: between different budgets
2. Geographical priority-setting: between regions and localities
3. Service priority-setting: between main areas of health care work
4. Treatment priority-setting: between types of treatment
   (a) for the same condition
   (b) for different conditions
5. Individual priority-setting: between individuals

structured; on the inclusionary pressures in clinical work; on the evaluation of health care; and on the principles and practice of resource allocation priority-setting. In order to explore these issues further I start by looking at some examples of clinical interventions which illuminate the structuring of demand and supply, as well as highlighting some of the problems of evaluating health care and of priority-setting.

The structuring of demand and supply

Hip replacements

I have chosen the example of the surgical replacement of the hip joint for a number of reasons. It is an example of a successful medical innovation that commands widespread support and for which demand is high; it is also an example of an intervention that deals with what would otherwise be a set of chronic problems associated with hip degeneration rather than a life-threatening condition; it is, however, an operation that is relatively expensive so demand within the NHS outstrips supply and there are waiting-lists. It is also an example of a medical remedy to a health problem where need increases with age, as is typical of many health problems, and this raises important issues about priorities.

A successful operation to replace a hip joint was first carried out in Britain in 1972 following work on replacement hip joints during the previous decade (Porter 1999: 623). The surgeons were responding to a pre-existing health problem—the incapacities, pain, and impaired mobility associated with hip degeneration—and once they could show that the operation was successful in reducing pain and increasing mobility, this success generated enormous service demand. The operation was clearly of benefit both to patients, and to the surgeons and the wider medical profession whose reputations were enhanced. For the profession it became a medical success story which affirmed the value of new medical technologies and of the profession's skills, expertise, and legitimacy. For patients it provided relief from long-term pain, suffering, and immobility at the price of the short-term pain and discomfort of major surgery and a somewhat longer period of recuperation.[5] Before this, those with hip degeneration had to cope with the pain themselves, perhaps with the support of some pain-relieving medicines, and to accept the resultant incapacity and immobility. As their condition deteriorated they might have to walk with the aid of a stick, end up in a wheelchair, or perhaps even be confined to their bed.

This example is illuminating in terms both of the structuring of the demand for health care and of its supply. The introduction of the hip replacement operations provides, in many respects, a straightforward example of how service demands are generated through the development of new medical technologies which cater for pre-existing health problems, a process that we can portray in terms of the simple model set out in Figure 6.1.

The term 'health problem' refers here to some problem of body or mind which may cause pain, suffering, or impaired functioning or make death more likely, and has an independent existence and material reality.[6] It is more or less interchangeable with the term 'health need', though neither is a very precise concept. The term 'health remedies' refers to interventions and treatments developed as ways of alleviating particular health problems, typically by professional healers, though a remedy may be developed by informal healers based on their own knowledge and expertise. The model indicates that health care demands are a product of two factors, health problems and the health remedies that are supplied by professionals (or lay people) to deal with them—in this case hip replacements. It shows how medical innovations structure health care demands, which may be articulated either by patients once they learn about the new innovation or by clinicians.

In the case of hip replacements the demand generated by the new procedure has been very considerable, and it is easy to see how medical innovations like this have contributed to the increase in the demands on health services over the postwar period. The numbers of hip replacement operations per annum has increased significantly since the operation was introduced in 1972, with the figures continuing to rise during the 1990s. In 1995–6, in the NHS in England alone, some 65,638 hip or 'head of femur' replacement operations were carried out (DOH 1996) and probably around a further 11,000 in the private sector.[7] The total annual cost to the NHS is very considerable, even though not all the demand is being met. The cost of an initial hip operation is roughly around £4,000 including consultations, hospital stay, physiotherapy, and check-ups, though prostheses vary considerably in price. For second (revision) operations

Figure 6.1 The demand for health care

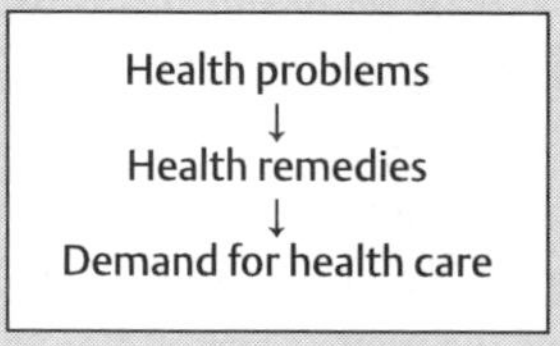

Health problems
↓
Health remedies
↓
Demand for health care

(necessary if the prosthesis wears out, as they can do after ten or fifteen years, or if the first operation is unsuccessful), the cost is around £10,000, since these operations are much more difficult.[8] With around one in ten operations currently revision operations, this makes the total annual NHS cost in England alone something in the order of £300 million out of the total NHS spending in the UK of some £43 billion (ONS 1999).

The statistics also show how, as we might expect, the distribution of hip replacement operations is positively related to age, since the chances of hip degeneration increase with age. The majority of the NHS operations in England, 77 per cent in 1995–6, were carried out on persons aged 65 and over, with 47 per cent performed on those aged 75 or more (DOH 1996), though precisely how far supply matches need is more debatable.[9] One important consequence is that, given the marked gender differences in longevity, far more women than men have hip replacements—more than double across all ages and more than treble amongst the 75s and over (DOH 1996). The age profile of those having a hip operation reflects an overall pattern in the NHS where much health care spending is concentrated on the elderly. This age profile is significant for two reasons. First, because gains in longevity, which mean a higher proportion of older people in the population, are likely to lead to an increase over time in patient demand for the operation; and second, because it raises the question of how high a priority should be placed on meeting the health needs of the elderly in comparison with other groups. Although most hip replacements are carried out on those aged 65 and over, many still have to wait for their operation, and face pain and suffering while they do so, as well as further deterioration of their hips, which makes the subsequent operation more difficult and more expensive. I look at the issues of age and priority-setting further below. For the moment it is important to note that, since hip replacements only last for a finite period (they should last ten years and may last twenty), the benefits of the operation need to be assessed over a reasonably short period.

The example of hip replacements also raises other issues about the structuring of supply. Faced with Muir Gray's question: 'Are we doing the right things?', the answer in the case of hip replacement operations is almost certainly yes. This is for two main reasons. First, the operation is typically very effective in that it reduces pain and suffering and improves mobility, and the associated risks are relatively small.[10] Significantly in this case, such a claim is not primarily dependent on careful, scientific double-blind trials—the preferred scientific strategy for evaluation—but primarily on clinical observations which simply compare the health outcomes of those who have had operations with those who have not (Nuffield Institute for Health Care 1996).[11] Hip replacements are also a relatively cost-effective or efficient intervention when compared with other medical interventions even though the replacements have a limited life-span, and there is controversy over the relative merits of different prostheses.[12] Second, it seems likely that there is a reasonably satisfactory match between the need for a hip replacement and supply, so that though some people have to wait for the operation, they tend only to be given to those with a clear need and probably few are carried out unnecessarily or inappropriately. This is in part because the identification of cases requiring treatment is relatively unproblematic. It is true that the level of hip replacements varies considerably across localities (the 10 per cent of health authorities that do the most replacements carry out twice as many as the 10 per cent who do the least (Klein et al. 1996: 67)). But some of this difference will be due to the different populations with a different spread of hip problems. Some will be due to differences in GP referral levels (which may be linked to the availability of specialists), some to differences in specialists' decision-making (including some who may decide to operate somewhat prematurely), and some to the length of waiting-lists. Nonetheless, if there is a problem it is almost certainly a problem of shortage of provision rather than over-supply in relation to health needs.

The one note of caution that needs to be sounded in relation to this medical success story relates to the issue of prevention. Doctors, whose main task is to deal with sick individuals, have focused their attention on dealing with hip degeneration once it has occurred. They have given far less attention to trying to prevent it. Recent attention to osteoporosis and to the claims that osteoporosis in women can be prevented or reduced through the use of hormone replacement therapy (HRT) has changed the picture a little. However, this preventive strategy has two important limitations. First, as a form of clinical prevention it involves direct medical intervention, rather than adopting a public health or even health promotion focus that attention to exercise and diet would involve.[13] Second, it tends to ignore issues of cost-effectiveness and the risks associated with this type of long-term, preventive drug therapy. HRT involves expensive medication from the time a woman reaches the menopause perhaps for the rest of her life, medication that has not been adequately evaluated on a lifetime basis.[14] There are, therefore, even in the case of hip replacements, some grounds for concern about whether public health and health promotion should have a higher priority on the supply side.

Tonsillectomies

The surgical removal of the tonsils as a treatment for repeated bouts of tonsillitis provides an illuminating contrast with hip replacements, primarily because this operation raises key questions about effectiveness. In this case the operation has a longer history going back to the last century, and played a central role in the growth of surgery in the first half of the twentieth century

(Howell 1995: 61–2). Tonsillectomy became one of the most common operations in hospitals in the 1920s and 1930s, and was still being carried out very widely in the 1950s and 1960s, even though the operation was painful and the cost to the NHS considerable. Again, this is a case of a medical innovation generating its own demand, with doctors recommending tonsillectomies for a broad range of tonsil problems, especially in children. However, as with many other medical interventions, the operation had not been evaluated very extensively. Indeed, tonsillectomy was one of A. L. Cochrane's examples in his path-breaking study, *Effectiveness and Efficiency* (1972). Cochrane bemoaned the lack of concern for issues of effectiveness and efficiency within medicine, and was particularly concerned that the effectiveness of some widely used treatments, including tonsillectomy, had not been adequately assessed. He commented that, though it had passed its peak, tonsillectomy was still then the commonest cause of admission of children to hospital in Britain, accounting for about 150,000 admissions per year.

In Cochrane's view the frequency with which tonsillectomy was carried out extended well beyond the desirable limits of its known efficacy. He points out that some limited attempts had been made to evaluate the operation using randomized control trials (RCTs), but there had been no proper attempt to compare surgical intervention with good medical care as opposed to simply doing nothing, and the assessment of efficacy was made on parental reports (in an era when parents usually believed the operation to be effective). Having reviewed the limited evidence, Cochrane concluded that that data suggested tonsillectomies were not very effective and were being carried out far too frequently. He called for better RCTs to assess their efficacy and urged that meanwhile:

> No case should be placed on a surgical waiting-list but always referred for medical treatment, and only when this fails after a prolonged trial should the case be sent to the surgeon. This should reduce the numbers of tonsillectomies to about one-fifth of the present numbers. (Cochrane 1972: 61)

It is essential to note that Cochrane did not reject the use of tonsillectomies altogether but called for them to be used far more cautiously. This is crucial because, whilst his text has often been read, correctly, as making a call for more studies of effectiveness, what is often ignored is the fact that his analysis indicates very clearly that *we cannot simply describe specific treatments as effective or ineffective*. The key issue concerns the effective *use* of treatments, that is for precisely what degree or form of the illness is the treatment effective. Yet the approach to evaluation often seeks to assess a treatment's effectiveness in general terms. This applies, for instance, to the evaluation of drugs tested on those with a particular illness. The objective in such testing is to establish that the drug has therapeutic benefits for the illness in question when compared with a placebo or some alternative medication. It is not to determine for exactly which degrees or forms of the disease, or groups of patients, the drug is effective. Yet it is precisely this that we need to know if drugs are to be used appropriately.

One way of portraying Cochrane's analysis is in terms of a continuum of tonsil problems from the mild to the severe. What had happened was that the threshold for intervention had come to be set far too close to the mild end of the spectrum, whereas the data indicated that the operation should only be considered in severe cases. This is shown in Figure 6.2, where the downward arrow on the left points indicatively to the boundary of the extensive range where the operation was carried out and on the right to the boundary where Cochrane believed intervention would be appropriate. The space between the arrows indicates the terrain of unnecessary or inappropriate treatment, the terrain where cases had been mistakenly identified as suitable for surgical treatment. For Cochrane the task was to narrow the use of tonsillectomies down to the restricted set of cases not amenable to other forms of treatment. A similar diagram could be used to portray the situation in terms of types of tonsil problem, raising the specific question of whether some forms of tonsillitis are more resistant to other types of treatment and more likely to require surgical intervention. The model could also be used to analyse the effectiveness of treatment for different patient groups. In this case the question would be whether, for instance, patients of a different age are more likely to recover without an operation.

Whereas the case of hip replacements suggests that supply is more or less in line with need or, if anything, does not meet the level of need, the case of tonsillectomies reveals how the development of a particular remedy came to generate a demand that was shown to outstrip need once its value was more carefully assessed. In thinking about the provision (supply) of health care we therefore need a more complex model than that set out in Figure 6.1 in which

Figure 6.2 Tonsil problems and tonsillectomies

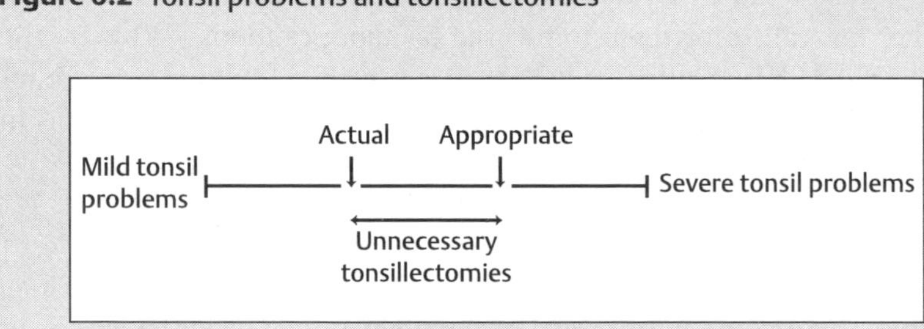

health remedies were seen simply as responses to pre-existing health needs and there was an assumption of some symmetry between health needs and health demands when a suitable treatment was developed. Such a model needs to include factors that encourage the use of treatments apart from health needs such as professionals' interests and those of commercial companies involved in the provision of treatment—suppliers of equipment and drugs—factors that I discuss further below. A more complex model is set out in Figure 6.3.

Since the 1960s the numbers of tonsillectomies being carried out has declined which might indicate that Cochrane's claims about the excessive use of tonsillectomies may have had some effect. However, it is difficult to determine how far this is so, and how far the decline is due to the development of new and more exciting forms of surgical intervention which began to occupy the interests and energies of surgeons.

Premature baby units

Another interesting example in relation to the impact of new medical technologies on demand for, and supply of, health care, and to issues of effectiveness, is intensive care for premature babies. In this case we can see a process in which the boundaries of what constitutes a health care problem are changed as medical technologies develop, as well as a lack of clarity as to what constitutes effectiveness.

The normal gestation period of babies is forty weeks, and until the 1950s babies born more than two or three weeks prematurely were unlikely to live. During the 1950s the growing use of incubators meant babies born even at thirty weeks might survive. The use of ventilators pushed this figure back further in the 1970s and since then new drugs and survival techniques, including improved ventilators, new forms of monitoring, and new drugs, have extended the period of possible foetus viability to twenty-three weeks if the baby is given intensive care in a specialist premature baby unit. The cost of

Figure 6.3 The supply of health care

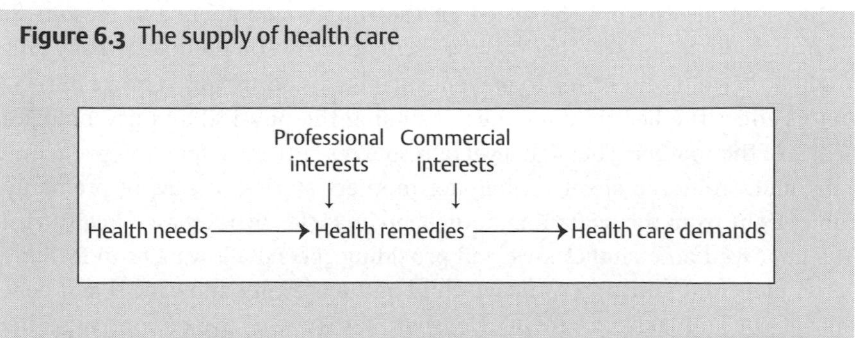

these units is high since they are very labour-intensive and require specialist nursing staff, both important factors in accounting for the rising cost of health services in the postwar period.

Until these innovations, it was taken for granted that babies born much before term would not survive. There would be pain and sorrow when the premature baby inevitably died, but hardly even a perception that there was a 'health' problem to be remedied. Now expectations that a very premature baby might survive are generated and its death seems less inevitable and so perhaps even harder to cope with. To many this would seem an acceptable price for the improved chances of survival for those who have the misfortune to have premature babies and a positive sign of technological advance. However, the issue of measuring the effectiveness of medical interventions in this context is particularly interesting. One of the most common indicators of effectiveness is survival. For example, the standard measure in assessing cancer treatments is to look at five-year survival rates, and the temptation is to apply this measure to premature baby units. Judged on this criterion the units are effective, since they do increase the chances of a premature baby surviving. However, against this marker of effectiveness, and indeed against the misery of the death of a premature baby, has to be set the fact that premature birth is associated with much higher levels of handicaps than full-term births, the level increasing the more premature the baby, with figures indicating that up to one half of babies born at twenty-three weeks will be brain-damaged (mainly due to oxygen shortage at critical times). It could therefore be argued that for the parents, pleasure at the infant's survival may be tempered by the subsequent difficulties they encounter as a result of any handicaps or by the problems for the child itself. Of course, it could be argued that the premature infant has the right to life and doctors and nurses must strive to maintain life even at great expense. Yet the pursuit of survival at shorter and shorter periods of human gestation is surely something that needs to be called into question and is surely a candidate for comparative evaluation to establish whether resources would be better deployed on alternative forms of clinical work.

Questions also need to be asked on the supply side about the reasons for premature birth, and whether the resources now used on premature baby units might be better spent trying to prevent such births occurring. A range of social factors affect the health of a foetus, including the physical and psychological health of the mother. The high level of resources currently spent on premature baby units could be spent on helping mothers at risk of having premature babies right from the beginning of their pregnancies by increased health visiting, improved antenatal classes, and providing special allowances to facilitate better diets and nutrition (we have child and maternity allowances and benefits but not a pregnancy benefit). However, for some of the reasons suggested in the previous chapter, medicine tends to concentrate on high technology solutions which bring prestige, status, and greater financial rewards, rather than the less dramatic, more routine work of supporting the physical and psychological health of pregnant women before they give birth.

Prozac

An equally controversial and illuminating example of the generation of patient demand from a very different part of the medical spectrum is provided by the introduction of Prozac for the treatment of depression. Prozac, a selective serotonin reuptake inhibitor (SSRI), was developed by Eli Lilly in the US and was first licensed by the US Food and Drug Administration in 1987. The new drug, which was initially used mainly for patients with severe, usually psychotic, depression, had the advantage over the tricyclics then dominant of working more quickly and having fewer side-effects. However, it became clear that Prozac had most impact on those with less severe forms of depression and also helped individuals to cope with stress and made them feel more positive about their lives (Kramer 1994). As a result, the drug began to be used for a far wider range of psychological conditions and for people who wanted the sense of positive wellbeing it was reputed to bring. Here we can see that in developing the new drug the company was responding to a perceived market opportunity arising from an established health problem—severe depression. However, in the process of introducing the drug the boundaries of the problem it was held to treat began to change: from severe to milder depression and then to stress and to personality attributes relating to self-esteem and self-confidence. And in the process of attracting new patients new health problems were generated altogether and demand was amplified. Indeed, the metaphor I introduced in Chapter 1 of a stronger and stronger medical microscope exposing a new range of health problems not visible before hardly seems apposite here, since what seems to have happened with Prozac is less that a new treatment lowered the threshold of what counts as depression, but that it has changed the nature of the gaze altogether and, with the active encouragement of the drug company, has constructed a new type of health problem where none existed up till then—and the same applies to the example of the survival of very premature babies.[15]

The term 'pathologization' describes this process of changing the boundaries of health problems rather better than the more common term 'medicalization', since the latter term has often been taken to suggest an active medical imperialism, whereas in this case, as in some others, the role played by the pharmaceutical companies is just as, if not more, important than that of the medical profession. The media have termed Prozac a 'lifestyle' drug, a label which neatly captures the fact that in many cases its use has little to do what was formerly constituted as ill-health; yet new drugs like these do change the boundaries of normal and acceptable bodily and psychological states, sometimes with unfortunate consequences.

This pathologization of what would before have been considered normal and outside the boundaries of health problems has profound implications for health services since it brings so many people into the pool of potential patients. One writer suggests, for example, that the broad category of what is termed 'affective spectrum disorder' (ASD), for which Prozac might be a suitable treatment, a disorder whose boundaries were broadened as a result of the introduction of the drug, affected 'possibly one third of the population of the world' (quoted in Shorter 1997: 323). Following the introduction of Prozac, ASD became the fashionable diagnosis and was applied to half of all patients visiting a psychiatrist in the US by 1993. Given this enormous pool of affective disorder, the potential demand for Prozac is huge, not least because its effectiveness depends on continuing usage; it is also difficult to determine when the drug should be stopped, so many who start using it may end up as long-term users, making it likely that the drug will be prescribed almost on a preventive basis. Not surprisingly, writing in 1997, Shorter could point out that Prozac had by then become the second most widely prescribed drug in the world.

Does the extensive use of Prozac matter? Certainly the cost of this rather indiscriminate form of prescribing is very great, and one of the concerns has to be that on grounds of the severity of health need some of the conditions for which it is prescribed may not have a very high priority in comparison with life-threatening illnesses (see below). Furthermore, as with premature baby units, it is not clear that this type of drug treatment provides the best solution to the milder depression with which it is supposed to deal, let alone issues of self-confidence. There is a range of evidence, for instance, that non-psychotic depression has social causes. This does not mean that no attention should be paid to the biochemistry of depression or that psychotropic drugs have no effect on mental processes; rather it is to say that studies of causation which look beyond the immediate biochemical changes show the impact of what happens in people's lives on the development of depression. For example, depression is currently about twice as likely to occur in women as in men, and it is clear that the level of stress that women have to face and the presence or absence of social support makes a crucial difference to whether they become depressed (Brown and Harris 1978; Thoits 1995).[16] It might well be more cost-effective to focus on a depressed woman's social situation and to provide more support for them in dealing with the difficulties they face than simply prescribe an anti-depressant such as Prozac on a long-term basis (and greater support might generate benefits across the whole family). There is also the issue of side-effects. Prozac may not be addictive, though the addictive quality of both

Librium and Valium, the minor tranquillizers which came onto the market in the early 1960s, only began to emerge a decade later. However, notwithstanding the claims that it has comparatively few side-effects, some have already been identified, especially a reduction in sexual desire, and others may emerge.

Viagra

A similar blanket demand is now being generated in the US with the launch of Viagra, a pill for male impotence, following its licensing in March 1998. In the US the demand for this drug is already considerable, with two million prescriptions written in the first three months, and like Prozac it is being termed a lifestyle drug. The British Government has been considering whether to include it on the list of drugs that can be prescribed on the NHS, though the potential cost is enormous, and has permitted its use only in the treatment of impotence arising from a restricted list of clearly defined medical conditions.[17] This cautious approach is not surprising given the potential cost to the NHS. Each tablet costs around £5 and one source estimates that there are two and a half to three million male impotence sufferers in Britain (*The Guardian*, 27 June 1998). Limited trials have also begun on the use of the drug for women, and there is talk of a potentially high demand from them. Such estimates may be exaggerations, but what is striking is that, whilst impotence is a long-recognized health problem for which some medical treatments were available, it was not formerly considered especially common.

The enormous demand for Viagra is apparently being produced by changing expectations and perceptions of what constitutes satisfactory sexual performance and what constitutes a health problem. It has generally been accepted that male potency often declines with age, and that this is usually inevitable; however this acceptance, albeit perhaps reluctant, is now being challenged by the belief that it is possible with new drugs for male potency to be restored. Moreover, there are fears that there will be a high demand from those who wish to enhance their potency and sexual pleasure—which formerly might well have been regarded as adequate. The extent of the initial demand suggests that men find any decline in potency difficult if not threatening, bound up as it is symbolically with conceptions of masculinity and male power, and faced with the chance to improve potency are changing their ideas of what is acceptable (whether their desire for greater potency is shared by their wives and partners is an interesting question). Certainly, to the increased risk of heart attacks, which are said to be one of the effects of the drug (and increased risks of headaches and blurred vision), should be added the possible negative as well as positive implications for sexual relationships so far little discussed.

There have been some studies of the causes of the types of male impotence formerly brought to medical attention, and some are undoubtedly physiological including the effect of other illnesses. Amongst possible physiological causes are the side-effects of other drugs, and there is a considerable irony in the fact that one 'wonder drug', Prozac, is said to reduce sexual desire, whilst another, Viagra, is designed to deal with that very problem. This generates a nightmare scenario, which already arises in some instances, of widespread polypharmacy with the multiplication of the drugs being taken by individuals, new ones being added to counter the effects of others, and little systematic assessment of what such drug cocktails do to body or mind.[18] Moreover, some causes, especially of the less severe problems of male impotence now being brought to attention as a result of Viagra, are undoubtedly socio-psychological and might be better dealt with through greater discussion of the individual's personal and sexual relationships.

What conclusions particularly pertinent to priority-setting can we draw from this discussion of specific examples of clinical interventions? Above all we can see how the demand for clinical interventions is shaped not only by pre-existing health needs but also by the development of health remedies, remedies which may come to be demanded and used well beyond the boundaries of their value. This is because their development and use are shaped not just by the presence of health problems but also by the activities, interests, and skills of professionals and medical companies (as well as by the media and patient groups). Demand should not therefore be regarded as an adequate measure of health needs or of the value of the treatment to the case or cases in question. Whilst professionals undoubtedly help the sick and do much valuable work, they also change perceptions and generate new demands not all of which can or should be met.[19] Indeed, there is a tendency for clinicians to concentrate on work that enhances their own professional interests as well as benefiting their patients and for them to be very free in their use of health care remedies. This situation is exacerbated by the strong commercial pressures on doctors encouraging them to use new technologies and new drugs. Consequently, whether we look at the shaping of demand or of supply we are faced with a central question of the extent to which clinical interventions are used in ways that meet health needs. I want to explore this area further by considering the inclusionary pressures that often lead clinicians to use treatments somewhat unselectively despite resource constraints. I then look further at the evaluation of clinical interventions.

Inclusionary pressures

It is clear from the examples discussed above that treatments developed for a particular range of cases often end up being used far more widely than originally envisaged. It might be argued that this is desirable, and is a measure of the reasonable access that many now do have to valuable medical treatments. Certainly, good access to medical treatments where they are needed is highly desirable. Nonetheless, it is clear that there are many examples of treatments that are used very freely, and a strong case can be made that they are often used too freely. Medical history is littered with treatments that became fashionable and were used very extensively at great cost in terms both of direct resources and the associated risks either for the individual or the wider population, only for it to emerge that their value in many cases was limited. Antibiotics are an obvious candidate. These undoubtedly offer an effective treatment for a range of serious conditions such as pneumonia; equally there is plenty of evidence of overuse, not least the development of antibiotic-resistant bacillae. This is because antibiotics are often used despite clear clinical contraindications (such as evidence that the illness is due to a virus against which they are ineffective, or that the illness is mild and the individual would recover without any treatment). Electro-convulsive therapy (ECT) is another example, introduced as a treatment for a wide range of severe mental disorders including schizophrenia and very widely used in the 1950s and 1960s, it was gradually shown only to have value in certain specific forms of depression when other possible remedies had been exhausted (Clare 1980). Radical mastectomy as a treatment for breast cancer was established after careful controlled trials to be no more effective than much more restricted tissue removal, yet though it is now being used a little more cautiously, it is still quite widely used on older women. Other possible candidates for treatments used too extensively are hormone replacement therapy, Caesareans, and tranquillisers, as well as drugs to prevent ulcers and high blood pressure when modifications to diet and exercise could be just as effective.

However, we need to distinguish a number of aspects to the claim that many clinical treatments are overused. The first is that in many cases recovery is likely without treatment or that alternative interventions, perhaps non-medical, would be just as effective. This is clearly an issue very pertinent to priority-setting. Of course, against this it might be argued that it is difficult to determine which individuals will recover without treatment or with the cheaper form of treatment. However, Cochrane's argument is that in such cases other treatments should be tried first and only if they fail should the more radical and more costly treatment be considered. The second aspect is that the dangers and risks associated with particular treatments may be overlooked in the enthusiasm for their use, and this is particularly important when an illness is less severe. With severe illnesses it is somewhat more likely that the potential benefits outweigh the risks; with less severe illness the balance of the equation often changes. The third is a claim that the widespread use of clinical interventions takes attention away from the crucial issue of taking prevention seriously.

The tendency to overuse treatments is the result of a phenomenon that I call 'clinical inclusion'. The problem is that the key boundaries with which clinicians have to operate are frequently far from clear-cut or precise. It is often difficult for a clinician to know whether a particular individual needs a specific treatment or not. Faced with the problem of setting exact boundaries on health needs, there are enormous pressures on clinicians to settle these boundary difficulties by inclusion, viewing individuals who consult them as having some health problem rather than none, providing them with treatment rather than excluding them, and using the latest, most sophisticated (and often most expensive) treatment rather than something simpler and cheaper. What this means is that a new treatment, which may be effective for a highly selected group of patients, begins to be used far more extensively than was originally envisaged and than is desirable.

One source of evidence of the lack of precision in boundary-setting is provided by the considerable variation that exists in the use of particular treatments and in GPs' levels of referral to specialist services (Farrow and Jewell 1993). I have already noted that hip replacement rates in some areas are double those of others, and the same study showed much larger differences for some other operations. For instance, the 10 per cent of health authorities with the highest rates of coronary artery bypass graft performed eight times as many operations as the 10 per cent with the lowest rates (Klein et al. 1996: 67). Partly this is due to the different patient populations and different priorities, but it is clear that much of the variation arises from different assessments of treatment needs, including which cases require specialist care, and of the enthusiasms, interests, and skills of consultants. In the US, for example, studies have shown that the percentage of women receiving hysterectomies varies sixfold between localities, a situation exacerbated by the financial incentives to be obtained from doing the operation. But even where there are no direct financial incentives very significant differences arise.

The pressures on clinicians to settle boundary difficulties inclusively rather than exclusively come from a number of different sources. In the first place, there is the imbalance of risk in the situations of uncertainty that typically characterize clinical work. As Thomas Scheff (1963) argued in the 1960s, clinicians are concerned about two types of error. First, that they will mistakenly diagnose a sick individual as healthy when the person in question does in fact have an illness, or not give them treatment when they would benefit from it. Second, that they will wrongly diagnose a healthy individual as sick when they are not, or give a treatment when it is not necessary. Of the two types of error the first carries potentially far greater risks in medicine (though Scheff contended that this did not apply to psychiatry and judgements of mental illness).[20] The individual could, for instance, die without treatment because of the clinician's mistaken belief that there was nothing wrong, whereas to give some treatment to a healthy individual will usually have less severe consequences even if the procedure carries some risks and is unpleasant. Consequently doctors tend to err on the side of caution and in situations of uncertainty diagnose illness and offer treatment—a tendency exacerbated by the increasing focus in medicine (and elsewhere) on controlling risks. In this context the risks of litigation, which have been a strong factor influencing medicine in the US for a number of years, and are now increasing in Britain, also encourage clinicians to engage in defensive medicine—that is, acting on inclusionary rather than an exclusionary basis, for instance, by carrying out many tests in the effort to ensure that absolutely nothing has been missed.

Second, the pressure towards clinical inclusion is strengthened by a further medical belief—a strong commitment to the value and importance of early treatment. There is widespread evidence that with many illnesses, most obviously many cancers, the chances of success are higher if treatment begins early before the problem has become too severe and relatively intractable. Whilst the evidence of the value of early treatment for many illnesses is incontrovertible, the belief provides an important rationale for setting the boundaries of illness quite widely, for not focusing exclusively on severe cases, and in situations of uncertainty including rather than excluding marginal cases.

Third, patients' demands also encourage clinical inclusion rather than exclusion. Once new treatments are introduced patients may, as I have argued, often expect or demand access to them, assuming they will be useful in their particular case, a situation often reinforced by media reports and the activity of medical companies and users' groups. It is widely noted that patients seem to want a prescription when they visit their GP and regard the encounter as unsatisfactory if they do not receive one. For patients a prescription provides a validation of their visit and makes it seem useful rather than a waste of time; it also provides a visible legitimation of their sickness and may be valuable in domestic and work contexts to achieve entry into the sick role. For GPs writing a prescription demonstrates their expertise and authority in the face of pressures on their time, and is frequently quicker and easier than explaining why a prescription is not necessary or considering alternatives. It helps to sustain a positive interaction between patient and doctor and provides a convenient ending to the consultation (Abel-Smith 1994: 122). The fact that a high percentage of prescribed drugs are never taken by patients is itself suggestive that many have been prescribed unnecessarily, though some would undoubtedly have been beneficial if they had been taken.

Fourth, financial arrangements may create incentives to encourage clinical inclusion rather than exclusion. This can arise when clinicians have a direct financial interest in treatment, for instance, when they are paid on a fee-for-service basis. For example, fee-for-service has been the basic method of payment for NHS dentistry since 1948 (apart from children's dental services), and for some GP services. Within dentistry the issue of unnecessary treatment generated sufficient concern in the 1980s that a committee was set up to report on the matter. It decided that a full investigation of the extent of such treatment was not needed, arguing that 'the vast majority do not undertake widespread and deliberate unnecessary treatment' (DHSS 1986: 21), a carefully qualified statement that actually accepts that the majority of dentists sometimes carry out unnecessary treatment, the authors observing that some dentists had 'the motive and opportunity to prescribe unnecessary treatment' (p. 25). The problem was sufficiently serious ('significant' in their words) for the committee to make a range of specific recommendations to detect and control it.

Fifth, there are pressures on clinicians from commercial medical and pharmaceutical companies to make use of their treatments and diagnostic screening devices—pressures to which there is often little resistance because of the value to the profession itself of any expansion in its therapeutic armoury. Many of the new technologies are of value if used selectively, but a new development may be presented as having more therapeutic benefits than is the case, or new equipment and instruments as more useful than they are. Doctors, as well as the commercial companies, stand to gain from over-optimistic assessments of the value of new treatments. Given the interdependence of the medical profession and medical companies, there is too little pressure on either to work out the precise limits of the value of particular interventions, so overuse and clinical inclusion are encouraged. In this context it is important to emphasize the point that diagnosis (boundary-setting) is often influenced by treatment decisions rather than diagnosis determining treatment as the theory suggests and the availability of new treatments changes diagnostic practices.[21]

Sixth and finally, there is the heroic, life and death culture that surrounds health and health care, which is often encouraged by the medical profession and is reinforced by the media. This not only automatically surrounds almost any aspect of health care with a favourable halo, but also portrays medical innovations and technologies as part of the battle of humankind against the enemy, disease. Consequently the culture not only encourages the search for new medical treatments (which is of course important) but also undermines critical thinking about the value of new treatments and encourages clinical inclusion.

Regrettably these difficult boundary-setting issues get too little explicit attention and are usually left for doctors to settle on a case-by-case basis. Faced with a woman who has read that HRT can be of value during the menopause and beyond, it is difficult for a doctor to turn round and say that it is not necessary for her, or that the treatment should only be used very selectively since there is little in the way of definitive guidance to back such an assertion in this particular case. The danger is that the doctor–patient relationship will be undermined by refusal to prescribe HRT, and there are few incentives to support such a refusal, apart from the frustrating barrier of the lack of resources, reference to which may lead to accusations against the doctor of rationing. What is needed is to provide ways of ensuring that doctors do not use treatments when they will be of little value.

Clinical evaluation

Adequate evaluation of clinical interventions offers one prospect of controlling treatment overuse as well as being vital to priority-setting. Notwithstanding Cochrane's call for more assessments of effectiveness and efficiency and the progress made since the publication of his text, there is still a great need for more extensive evaluations of health interventions, particularly assessments that do not simply attempt an overall assessment of a specific treatment but refine that evaluation in relation to three dimensions: the form of the illness, its severity, and patient characteristics. The need for more extensive evaluation to enable effective use can be clearly demonstrated in relation to drug treatments.

In many respects new drugs are subject to more systematic testing than other new medical treatments, as they have to be approved before they are put on the market. Tests of new drugs, as of other clinical interventions, focus both on efficacy and safety, since while a drug may be effective in, for instance, controlling a particular symptom, it may have severe side-effects, the acceptability of a new drug depending on the balance of therapeutic and side-effects. Tests follow the preferred scientific model of randomized control trials (RCTs), allocating individuals randomly to treatment and control groups, the control group against which the new drug is being compared receiving either a placebo or an alternative form of medication. In Britain tests on some of the patients must last at least a year, and overall at least 1,000 patients must have been involved in the trial of the new drug.[22]

Nonetheless, the testing of new drugs is arguably not as extensive as it should be. One of the problems is that the length of time over which testing has to occur is very limited, yet adverse side-effects may only emerge after use over a long period of time or the problem may only be visible in the offspring of those who have been taking a particular medication. The latter occurred with thalidomide, which was prescribed to pregnant women to control morning sickness but was eventually proved to have teratogenic effects producing defects in the embryo, which lead to multiple handicaps in the children who were born (*Sunday Times* Insight Team, 1980). Another problem is that drugs are tested only on selected samples. Usually they are only tested on adult men (women are typically excluded because of the dangers to any foetus), and the drug is then licensed for adults. The exclusion of women, though sensible, is a problem given metabolic differences and also because it means that there is no testing of possible consequences for the foetus. So, too, is the absence of any requirement for separate testing for the elderly, since they also have different metabolic levels from younger people. This was illustrated very dramatically by the case of Opren, an anti-inflammatory drug for the treatment of arthritis produced by Lilly, which was introduced onto the British market in 1980. After licensing the drug was shown to have toxic affects among the elderly, including dangers of liver failure, adverse skin reactions, and some carcinogenic properties, and one or two deaths occurred (Abraham 1995: ch. 4). The initial testing had not included any older patients, even though the drug was to be used to treat arthritis. More recently, concern has been expressed that drugs licensed for the treatment of adults are being widely used in the care of premature babies.

Another limitation of the samples used to test new drugs is that the patient groups are usually selected from persons with very definite cases of the illness which the medication is designed to treat. However, as I have already indicated, in clinical contexts the new treatment is likely to be used much more widely, often for those with less certain or less severe problems. Yet the treatment will rarely have been evaluated for its potential benefits and the associated risks across a highly diverse range of cases. New treatments need to be evaluated across a very broad spectrum of cases.

Another problem with drug evaluations is that commercial pressures encourage the pharmaceutical companies to read the results of trials in ways favourable to their products, and these readings are sometimes accepted by the bodies charged with advising on their licensing such as the Committee for the Safety of Medicine in Britain (and there have been some instances where results have been fabricated by companies). A further limitation of many trials is that there is little attempt to assess the interaction effects of one drug on another, though these can be considerable. Some interaction effects may be identified such as adverse effects if the drug is taken with alcohol (perhaps on the basis of clinical reports), but many others have not been examined. Significantly, too, the system of reporting adverse effects in clinical contexts is permissive not mandatory. Doctors in Britain are given yellow forms to report any adverse effects on patients to the Committee on the Safety of Medicines, but there is no requirement to report them.

Evaluation of other medical interventions is often even less adequate than that for drugs, not least because of the ethical problems associated with testing, as well as the problems of time and money. As clinicians doctors are expected to provide help and treatment for their patients, which militates against using them as subjects in treatment evaluations. Scientific assessment requires a focus on the potential long-term benefits of new treatments on populations, which may be at the expense of the interests of existing patients. The use of RCTs usually means withholding treatments that might be beneficial, as well as securing patients' informed consent to participation in the trial. Moreover, frequent modifications to new treatments make scientific evaluation more difficult.

There is now increased awareness of the paucity of clinical evaluations, and a number of strategies are being developed to deal with the problem. I want to focus on two: evidence-based practice and treatment protocols, and quality and clinical audit.

Evidence-based health care and treatment protocols

There has been a strong emphasis over the past decade on what is called evidence-based medicine or evidence-based health care. Cochrane's call in the early 1970s for a more adequate assessment of the effectiveness and efficiency of medical treatments had resonances with the neo-liberal call during the 1980s for greater effectiveness and efficiency in health care. However, the focus in the latter period was primarily on greater efficiency in the delivery of care and the avoidance of waste, to be solved by better management rather than on the need for a more critical evaluation of the content of health care itself. Yet this call for greater efficiency and effectiveness undoubtedly encouraged support for evidence-based medicine, which became the mantra of the 1990s.

Essentially the requirement of evidence-based medicine, a term first introduced in Canada towards the end of the 1980s, is that health workers should draw on the available research evidence in making clinical decisions. It calls for a particular approach to clinical work, 'a process of systematically locating, appraising, and using contemporaneous research findings as the basis for clinical decisions' (Rosenberg and Donald 1995). In that respect it makes explicit what was implicit in Cochrane's argument—that the evidence on effectiveness and efficiency once obtained should be used by clinicians in making their decisions. A new centre, named after Cochrane, was established in Oxford in 1992 to gather research on the efficacy of treatment and make it readily available to clinicians using information technology. There has also been a plethora of new publications reporting the findings of recent research to clinicians in an accessible form, as well as new, simpler ways of expressing the results of such studies. For example, effectiveness is now often expressed in terms of the number needed to treat (NNT)—i.e. the number of persons who have to be treated for there to be one successful outcome—and risk in terms of the number needed to harm (NNH)—the number who have to be treated for there to be a given adverse effect: for instance, how many women have to be given Caesareans for one to die.[23] There has also been pressure (and some new resources) to encourage clinicians to carry out their own research.

However, subscribing to the philosophy of evidence-based practice and putting it into operation routinely are very different matters, not least because if the ideal model is followed the actual use of evidence-based practice by individual clinicians can be difficult and time-consuming. Perhaps not surprisingly, there is evidence that its adoption is far less widespread than is suggested by the frequency with which the term is invoked (Walshe and Ham 1997). The ideal model requires the clinician not just to find out whether a particular treatment is typically effective or not, but also to assess its potential value for the particular patient—precisely what is needed if treatments are to be used only when they are likely to have some benefit. This involves having access to data on very precise clinical indications for its use, which may mean scrutinizing a number of different studies and is just the sort of systematic data on effectiveness that is often lacking. It may also mean withholding relatively ineffective treatments from patients, often difficult in the face of their demands. This suggests the need for guidelines or protocols on the use of specific treatments setting out clearly the clinical indications for their use. Such protocols, which are now being more widely developed, may take the form of step-wise decision trees, and may mean, as Cochrane advocated, that particular (often new and more expensive) treatments are only used if other (often cheaper) treatments have been tried and failed. They are also important in providing a clear rationale if doctors have to justify their decisions.

The recent focus on evidence-based care is reflected in the Government's decision to establish a new National Institute for Clinical Excellence (NICE). This will advise doctors on the best way to organize services and treat patients, and will make available data on effectiveness, including the provision of treatment protocols that specify the clinical indications for the use of particular treatments and the decision trees that clinicians should follow in making decisions about treatments. Such strategies are vital since they shift the focus to specifying the circumstances under which a treatment should be used.

Quality and clinical audit

The concern for adequate evaluation of clinical work is also being applied to the work of particular clinicians. Here the focus is not on assessing the effectiveness and efficiency of particular treatments but on the effectiveness and efficiency of particular clinicians, which is often discussed in terms of ensuring quality, though the term can be used in relation to both types of assessment. Practitioner performance is a very important issue, since in the wrong hands (which may mean inexperienced hands) an effective treatment may become very ineffective. Assessment of clinicians' work requires a different form of scrutiny and one which the medical profession at least has been especially reluctant to accept. (It may also require different organizational arrangements which ensure that difficult treatments are only carried out by highly trained specialists.) Part of the problem has been medicine's insistence on securing a high degree of professional autonomy and its consequent reluctance to accept external scrutiny, whether of the content of its work or of the performance of its practitioners. This autonomy has meant that its activities have not been subject to a high degree of external scrutiny, and the policing of standards and the ensuring of quality have been jealously guarded prerogatives of the profession itself. Even the challenges to medical authority over recent years have so far left much of its autonomy in this sphere intact.

Doctors are, of course, concerned about the quality of the work they carry out and have some formal mechanisms intended to ensure quality, such as the selection and training of new recruits—choosing the most suitable people and giving them the right knowledge and skills before they are accepted onto the medical register. Both are important, though one could question the selection criteria that operate (such as considerable recruitment from medical families) and the content of the training (the emphasis on biomedicine at the expense of social and psychological sciences). But initial selection and training are not sufficient. Mechanisms are also necessary once a doctor is trained to maintain high-quality practice, yet they have been limited. The NHS has introduced financial incentives to encourage doctors to attend courses in order to keep up to date with new developments. Moreover, as a result of the recent case against three medical employees of the Bristol NHS Trust arising from the very high death rates amongst infants undergoing heart surgery, the Government, with the backing of the General Medical Council, is making 'revalidation' of qualifications every five years mandatory. Up to now the main formal mechanism has been the threat of being struck off the medical register, but this device has largely been used to regulate *conduct*, not competence and performance. Summons to appear before the GMC usually result from allegations of sexual misconduct with patients, fraud, or a criminal conviction, not from clinical incompetence, and significantly those who are struck off are often reinstated relatively quickly. The narrow role played by the GMC was highlighted by the Bristol case which led to two doctors being struck off the register and was a rare exception in its focus on competence, and has prompted calls for better mechanisms to prevent doctors with such poor records continuing to perform operations.

The profession itself has tended to claim that neither external scrutiny nor further formal mechanisms are necessary to ensure adequate standards because there are sufficient informal mechanisms in place to achieve this end. They suggest that medicine operates as a collegial community which regulates the conduct of members, recognizing and detecting problems, such as a doctor with alcohol problems, and providing support for them including, if necessary, helping to ease the individual out. This scrutiny includes, they contend, poor performance and the provision of advice and support to ensure improvement. It is clear, however, that such mechanisms have not been adequate. The danger has always been that the medical club operates in a protective manner to defend the interests of the profession (to maintain their reputation for quality and the respect on which they depend) rather than to guarantee performance, which would be in the patients' interests. Any intervention, if it occurs, is often too little too late. In this context is significant that the medical Chief Executive of the Bristol NHS Trust knew of the poor operating record of his colleagues, but allowed them to continue with some operations.

A more recent mechanism for trying to ensure quality is medical audit. This has been defined as 'the attempt to improve the quality of medical care by measuring the performance of those providing that care, by considering the performance in relation to desired standards, and by improving this performance' (Marinker 1990: 3). Audit has considerable potential to improve standards. However, the value of clinical audit depends on the care and thoroughness with which it is carried out, the willingness of those carrying it out to make independent and, if necessary, critical judgements, and the uses to which the resulting data are put. There is a danger that medical audit will in practice mean not audit *of* medicine but audit *by* the medical profession. Yet while doctors should be involved in medical audit, others also need to be—managers and patient representatives. It is also vital that where problems are identified action should be taken to deal with them.

The concept of clinical audit has been extended and broadened in recent NHS policy documents which introduce the concept of clinical governance as:

> a framework through which NHS organisations are accountable for continuously improving the quality of their services and safeguarding high standards of care by creating an environment in which excellence in clinical care will flourish. (Secretary of State for Health 1998b: 33)

Such a framework should include 'a comprehensive programme of quality improvement activity (such as clinical audit and evidence-based practice)', 'clear policies aimed at managing risk', and 'clear lines of responsibility and accountability for the overall quality of clinical care' (Secretary of State for Health 1998b: 35, 38). However clinical governance will not in itself control the overuse of treatments or help in priority-setting without clear standards and precise protocols. Moreover, there are also important issues about the monitoring of doctors' performance, as the experience of assessing teachers' work indicates. The individual performance review model is likely to have many advantages over the publication of national league tables of hospital performance (though the Government has committed itself to publishing such tables).[24]

Determining resource allocation priorities

Recognizing the way demand and supply are structured by a range of forces in addition to health needs, the problems of clinical inclusion, and the need for more systematic clinical evaluation of clinical interventions, we can now consider how priorities can be set. Here the issue of comparison is placed centre stage. In looking at determining priorities between treatments and individuals three main criteria need to be included, each informed by different ethical considerations: health needs, health benefit and cost. I look at each in turn.

Health needs

Many would argue that health need should be the central criterion in allocating health care, and that those who are sickest have the greatest need for health care and should have the highest priority. Underpinning this criterion are the principles of justice and equity on which the NHS was founded: that services should be allocated on the basis of medical need, not the ability to pay. Of course, as I have already noted 'need' is as imprecise concept, but this does not mean that we can or should do without it (Doyal and Gough 1991). We routinely and regularly make assessments of need, including health needs, and it is essential that we retain some assessment of need in thinking about the provision of health care. I use the term 'health need' here to indicate an external assessment of the severity of a health problem. Certainly the level of health need has been an important principle in the allocation of resources between the main types of services within the NHS, and helps to account for the concentration of resources on acute services, and for the speedier access to health care in emergencies such as accidents, and for severe, life-threatening illnesses such as cancers. It accounts, for instance, for a Government statement that the waiting period for treatment for those with cancer should be not more than two weeks.[25] It has also been an important principle in the geographical allocation of resources and was embedded in the Resource Allocation Working Party formulae (1976) in the form of mortality and fertility rates as well as the age distribution of the different populations. It is now also a clear principle in individual priority setting. For example, it is explicit policy to target specialist mental health services on those with the severest problems—'the tip of the iceberg'—severity here often being assessed in terms of the level of danger to self and others (Audit Commission 1994: 5).

One difficulty with this criterion is measuring need. I mentioned earlier the importance of distinguishing between health problems and the demand for health care and patients' requests cannot be used as a measure of need. I also discussed the difficulty doctors have in setting the boundaries of illness and their inclusionary tendencies, which mean that if an individual comes with some health complaint they tend to assume need. However, we have to distinguish between agreeing a measuring-rod of need and the difficulties that may arise in judging individual cases, the former being easier than the latter. The usual indices of health need are the degree to which the problem is life-threatening or the amount of pain, suffering, and incapacity involved. However, it is also important to give explicit attention to the issue of chronicity as one dimension of need, since long-term problems have often been given lower priority within medicine than life-threatening ones. What is required is not to usurp the significance attached to the life-threatening, but rather to make sure that the duration of pain and suffering is brought into the equation. It is also important to note that the measurement of health needs can and should include knowledge of future health states as well as of present ones. Early treatment of many cancers can be judged highly desirable on the grounds of health needs alone since there is a clear, well-established trajectory for many of them. The same can also apply to preventive interventions if the risk of developing a particular illness can be clearly established and is high. There is, however, always a danger here, as there is with chronicity, that those with pre-existing, life-threatening problems take precedence over those who have not yet developed them, particularly where the risk is uncertain. Yet priority-setting must look at the health needs of those who are not yet sick as well as of those who already are.

Of course, applying agreed measuring-rods of severity to individual cases is more difficult, and the uncertainty that surrounds the judgement of cases is a major pressure towards clinical inclusion. Yet such judgements are routinely made and cannot be avoided.

Health benefit

The logic and importance of health needs in any consideration of priority-setting is simply that prima facie those in worst health should have the highest priority: those with cancer, heart disease, or severe injuries, have higher priority than those with varicose veins, relatively minor injuries, or, say, mild depression. However, whilst health needs should be central to geographical and service priorities and should be a *sine qua non* in the allocation of *care* and *support* to individuals—the sickest and most frail must be cared for—it cannot be the sole criterion with regard to the provision of *treatment*. It has to be balanced by a consideration of the likely benefit to be derived from treatment and of its cost. Here utilitarian considerations and issues of effectiveness enter the ethical picture. A major drawback of making health need the sole criterion for determining treatment priorities is that those with the severest problems may be hardest to treat effectively. I have already noted that a case can be made on grounds of health need alone for the value of the early treatment of severe illnesses, and this case is reinforced by consideration of health benefits, since the potential benefits may be greater if the illness is likely to prove incurable in its later stages, as can often be the case with cancer. Equally, treatment may actually be more expensive and difficult as the illness progresses. The same applies not just to the stages of one specific illness but to comparisons between illnesses. Some of the most life-threatening illnesses are hardest to treat, particularly if the individual has succumbed to numerous other health problems. Consequently, it is not clear that the sickest should always have priority in treatment allocation, and in some cases requiring someone to pass a threshold before they get access to an operation would be highly undesirable, if their condition would get worse and be harder to treat as a result. The assessment of the likely benefits resulting from particular treatments, both for specific degrees and forms of illness and for specific types of patient, do need to be brought back into the equation as the second consideration.

The key element added to health need through the introduction of the criterion of health benefit are the issues of whether the intervention is effective and necessary in the individual case. A remedy should only be used if there is evidence on the basis of past experience and/or scientific evaluation that it is likely to be an appropriate, necessary, and effective treatment *for the patient in question*. This means not just determining the efficacy of a treatment at the aggregate level, including the risks and side-effects, for a highly selected group of well-identified cases, but determining the appropriateness and potential value of the treatment for the particular individual. Would an alternative, less invasive procedure do the job just as well? Should other treatments be tried first and the particular treatment only used if they fail? Would the individual be likely to recover without treatment?

One tool devised by British health economists for comparing the health benefits of different treatments for the same or different illnesses is known as the Quality Adjusted Life Year or QALY. As a measure of health benefits the QALY incorporates two variables: the length of survival and the quality of that survival (which can vary over time). If, for instance, as a result of an operation a person survives but typically does so without any real consciousness or dignity, then this intervention is judged less effective than one where the same length of survival is achieved but the quality of life is far higher—a return to normal activities and so forth. If cost is further added to the equation, then treatments can readily be compared in terms of their cost-effectiveness.

However, the use of QALYs raises numerous problems. It may not be easy to identify clear, measurable outcomes of some interventions, not least because it is hard to identify specific interventions and specific outcomes—as with the long-term care for those with chronic illness. This may be one reason why QALYs have had a less extensive role in resource allocation priority-setting than might be expected.[26] There is also the difficulty of finding satisfactory measures of the quality of life. The most widely used indices have been physical mobility and level of distress, with pain as a key component of distress. These are measured in terms of the judgements of groups of individuals about particular states which are allocated a position on a scale from 0, death, to 1, normal health, with the possibility of scores below zero (states worse than death)—the choice of those involved in making the assessments affecting the outcome.

In addition to these practical methodological problems, there is also a major problem with the conceptual underpinnings of the QALY as an instrument for making comparisons. There are three related points. First, the instrument focuses on, and measures, health benefits making no assumptions about the value of improvements in health—it treats improvements in health which have an equivalent QALY as equal whether or not one person is seriously ill and the other is not. Put another way, there is no starting-point of evaluation of the level of medical need, so that the calculus may end up suggesting that we choose to enhance the health of those who are already fitter and ignore the ill-health of those who are sicker—an issue to which I return below.

The second major problem is that QALYs, like many measures of effectiveness, are usually used to compare treatments for particular diseases or conditions in an aggregate way. This assumes that specific treatments are either effective or not and ignores issues concerning the precise boundaries of their efficacy (are they only effective for severe cases?) and of how easy it is to identify the cases likely to benefit from treatment. Yet, as I have already argued, treatments may be effective for one range of cases and not for others—it is their effective use that is the issue.

Third, as QALYs incorporate the *length* of survival into the equation they are biased towards the young and against the elderly. The convention of using five-year survival to measure the effectiveness of clinical interventions is widespread and longstanding; it provides a very useful measure for comparing different treatments for the same life-threatening condition or when looking at improvements in the survival rates for particular illnesses over time, the convention of using RCTs ensuring that patient characteristics are held constant. However, when QALYs are used to compare different treatments *for different illnesses* survival data are given a different role. How long patients are likely to survive after the treatment becomes a criterion of whether the treatment for one type of illness should be given a higher priority than a treatment for a very different illness. And since different illnesses are associated with different patient groups this generates biases. For instance, treatments for conditions common in the elderly typically generate lower QALYs as their survival rates will frequently be lower, in part because age may increase the risks associated with the treatment, but more importantly because older people necessarily have shorter life expectancies than younger people. This does not mean that all treatments for conditions common in the elderly fare badly in QALY assessments once costs are taken into account—hip replacements generate a higher QALY than heart bypass operations even though the latter are typically carried out at younger ages, since heart bypass operations are very expensive and the subsequent chances of survival are not very good. Similarly there is also evidence that QALYs are biased against those in poorer social circumstances since these may adversely affect their chances of surviving an operation. Of course, discrimination against the elderly and other social groups in access to health care can occur without the use of measures such as QALYs, and there is plenty of evidence of such discrimination in health care—such as only routinely calling those under 65 for breast screening. However, QALYs makes such discrimination inevitable because of the importance given to length of survival in assessing health benefit when comparing treatments for different illnesses, and because there is no direct and explicit measure of health need, a criterion that need to be included as a counterbalance to biases against groups with poor health risks.

The defence for such highly contentious discrimination against the elderly is that in a situation of scarce resources it is more important to ensure the survival of the young than the elderly. The belief that this is the difficult if ultimately necessary choice that has to be made is grounded in longstanding ideas about the importance of restoring the productive or potentially productive (children) to health. It can also be sustained and supported by the elderly themselves, who sometimes claim that their medical needs should have lower priority (probably exacerbated by a generational tradition of not making demands on welfare services where possible). Yet it can be questioned on a range of grounds. One is that equity requires that all people regardless of age, sex, ethnicity, or social class should be treated equally in relation to need (and given an equal chance of treatment), which is why need is such an important criterion. Another is that elderly people have invested in society (and the majority of them in health services) and so should reap the benefits of that investment rather than be cast aside once their productive life is deemed over (one irony being that many individuals are required to leave the labour force and productive activity rather than choosing to do so). What is happening here is that a particular criterion of social worth, age, is being formally built into the determination of priorities. In this respect what can already happen in practice is in danger of being formally institutionalized.

To criticize the assumptions incorporated into QALYs does not mean that survival, quality of life, and effectiveness are not important in assessing health benefit. Rather, it is to say that they need to be viewed rather differently. First, when comparing treatments for different conditions the measuring-rod must include the chances of survival over a limited period—say six months or a year (though not the length of survival beyond that, as it is in the QALY measure of health benefit)—as well as the chances of reducing pain, suffering, or incapacity. Second, effectiveness needs to be determined in relation to specific degrees and forms of a health problem rather than in relation to broad categories of disease. And third, it must be considered in conjunction with health need.

Of course, potential health gains are not independent of health needs: in theory the sickest have potentially most to gain from receiving treatment and the least sick the least. However, health needs and health benefits do not necessarily coincide, as when sickness is so severe that little can be done for the individual other than to provide palliative care. Most would accept that doctors should not strive officiously to keep patients alive if survival would involve little more than being in a vegetative state, though there can be temptations and pressures to do so (unhappy and demanding relatives, uncertainty about whether further treatment might help, and so forth). It is important to note, however, that those with milder health problems will often be those where the health benefits will be smallest. Consequently the second criterion, like the first, frequently provides good grounds for giving lowest priority to those with the least severe problems. It does not, however, necessarily rule out giving priority to preventive work where the populations in question are healthy. The health gains from clinical prevention may be extensive—vaccinations are a case in point. So may the gains from health promotion, though its track record so far is not very good. And so, too, may the gains from public health interventions, and it is very important that all three types of preventive work are assessed for their health benefits. Indeed, there is almost certainly a strong case for greater investment in public health medicine.

A further consideration in assessing health benefits relates to the issue of the likelihood of health benefit. Treatments may have low levels of effectiveness even for highly selected cases, and we need to consider how good the chances have to be that a treatment will be of value for its use to be justified and for it to be given priority. If there is only a one in ten chance that it will work, is that enough? In part this will depend on the severity of the health problem, and a lower level of effectiveness may be justifiable if the problem is severe. This is, of course, where cost also starts to enter the picture. If a treatment is rarely effective but is inexpensive then its use may be justified if its side-effects are minimal. Where low effectiveness coincides with high costs and risks, then the treatment should surely have low priority except in very severe cases. However, it needs to be noted that the level of effectiveness does not necessarily remain constant over time; treatments can improve, and often need a period of development before they reach their full potential.

Cost

The third criterion, cost, is at first sight the most contentious, as it suggests it may be justifiable to deny people treatments because they are too expensive and gets us to the heart of controversies about rationing and priority-setting. Two points need to be made. First, in my view the extent of unselective use of treatments for people with low health needs, where the health benefits are also low, which results from the biases towards clinical inclusion, is considerable and its curtailment would reduce some of the demands on the NHS budget. This claim is controversial, and it is likely that some interventions for severe ilnesses currently in restricted use are highly effective and/or have fewer side-effects, and need to be used somewhat more widely even though they are expensive (possible candidates are Taxol in the treatment of ovarian cancers and Clozapine for the treatment of schizophrenia).[27] Second, others have argued that the emphasis on effectiveness and evidence-based medicine as a solution to the problems of priority-setting shows a misplaced confidence in science—a 'new scientism', and that whilst it 'offers great scope for improving the quality of medicine and health care', it is 'not a philosopher's stone for converting scarcity into plenty' (Klein et al. 1996: 104). However, my claim here is not that greater attention to the effectiveness and appropriateness of treatments will vitiate the need for priority-setting, but rather that the assessment of health benefits must be underpinned where possible by systematic data on effectiveness and also by protocols indicating criteria of appropriate use, and that such an approach would reduce the use of some treatments, particularly for less severe illnesses, and so save some resources.

Second, the inclusion of cost considerations is important notwithstanding efforts to increase NHS resources, precisely because whatever the success of these endeavours it will still not be possible to meet all health needs, given the way in which new treatments are emerging so rapidly and health expectations rising so markedly. Whilst it is tempting to believe that treatments should be made available regardless of cost, attention to costs can be helpful in thinking about the direction and character of health care. If, for instance, drug companies faced a regime where they not only had to show that drugs were effective and the range of their effectiveness, but also the value for money they offered, their work might be shaped in rather different ways. And the same applies to the activity of clinicians. It is surely desirable for there to be more work on low-cost solutions to the problems of, say, arthritis as against more work on highly expensive ways of reducing yet further the age at which premature babies can survive. The advantages to professionals of developing high-technology solutions need to be counterbalanced by greater attention to costs. It is important to note, too, that cost needs to be introduced as a factor in conjunction with consideration of health needs and likely health benefits rather than on its own. Treatments that have the lowest priority are those where the health needs fall lower down the scale, that are likely to lead to low health benefits because they are relatively ineffective, and that are also costly. In vitro fertilization, which is expensive, is not associated with life-threatening illness, and, where only a low percentage of treatments result in a pregnancy, almost certainly falls into this category.[28]

An interesting recent example that illustrates the importance of bringing costs into the equation is a consultant's call for women to be given the right to choose to have Caesareans if they want one without any reference to the cost of such a policy. The level of Caesarean births has increased markedly in the postwar period, from less than 4 per cent of births in 1958 to 13 per cent in 1992 (Treffers and Pel 1993), an increase that has been justified on the grounds of ensuring the survival of the infant when there are complications such as high blood pressure in the mother, though there are grounds for suggesting that Caesareans are already used excessively. The idea that women should be able to choose to have a Caesarean primarily for their own comfort and convenience, which would increase Caesarean levels yet further, almost certainly fails on all three criteria—the health need is minimal, the health benefit is small (and there are health risks), and the cost is significantly greater than for a normal pregnancy.

Priority-setting in practice

Introducing three clear criteria in setting priorities does not, of course, settle all areas of debate, not least because we have to determine the weights to be given to the respective criteria. Comparisons have to be made between very disparate health needs, on levels of effectiveness for the individuals in question where they are known, and on cost (what, for instance, is the level of health need for couples who find it difficult to conceive?). There are two key questions here. Should priorities be set locally or on a national basis? And who should set priorities?

There are three major reasons why some form of national framework is needed: equity, impact, and enforcement. In the first place, a national framework is more equitable. Local priority-setting provides enormous scope for inequities between localities. Such differences already exist and are sometimes referred to as 'rationing by postcode'. Whether you can secure in vitro fertilization on the NHS should not depend on where you live but on national priorities that have been agreed for the service. The construction of national guidelines also allows a single body such as the new National Institute for Clinical Excellence to collect and review the relevant evidence, which is likely to be a more efficient process than efforts to carry out such work across numerous sites. National priority-setting is also likely to facilitate the vetting of procedures across a broader range of cases. The political disadvantage for the government in setting national guidelines is that they will be associated with priority-setting and rationing. However, most people are already aware that the government determines the level of NHS resources and the advantages of explicit priority-setting are considerable.

Second, there is the issue of impact. So far the evidence indicates that local priority-setting tends to focus on making marginal changes and does not effect any major shift of resources. It allows the bulk of resource allocation to follow historic patterns and to be influenced by local factors, such as whether there is a specialist keen to develop a particular treatment, or a vocal pressure group backing a particular service. The theory underpinning the 1990 division between purchasers and providers in the NHS was that purchasers could set priorities and make purchasing decisions on a more rational basis. In practice, the changes were small. Some health authorities made decisions to exclude one or two procedures such as tattoo removal altogether; others required special authorization for treatments on a restricted list, and introduced criteria for eligibility for particular treatments or forms of care.[29] However, the limited nature of such endeavours so far means that the implicit rationing of the NHS based on clinicians' decisions has largely been retained. Whilst primary care groups may help to effect some shift from individual clinicians working out their own priorities, often on an ad hoc basis, to making collective judgements on priorities at the local level, the evidence from the work of health authorities in the 1990s suggests it will need more work at the national level to effect more radical changes.

A third, related point is that a national framework is important if priority-setting is to be enforced, since it offers the justification and authority for controlling health care practice that local health bodies are unlikely to have. On the one hand, protocols need to be well publicized, and it is easier to do this more effectively at a national level with a set of uniform guidelines. On the other hand, while enforcement will need to implemented at the local level, national powers can be used to prevent certain treatments being used too widely or being given too high a priority within the NHS (the restrictions on the prescribing of Viagra are a case in point). The need for some regulatory mechanism to ensure that clinicians follow the guidelines is also necessary on grounds of equity. This should mean that greater attention is given to using treatments when they are likely to prove effective and that there should be more regulation of the performance of individual clinicians and the quality of clinical practice.

As regards the question of who should make the decisions on resource allocation priorities, this must surely be a matter of open discussion and decision-making, with contributions from politicians, clinicians, health managers, and the public. I have already noted that lay judgements are incorporated into the quality of life assessments used in QALYs, but public views can also be used to aid in determining priorities in other ways. For example, 'citizens' juries' composed of groups of lay people have been used to determine treatment priorities. In order to aid their assessments the juries are given a range of information about effectiveness and cost by experts who put the arguments for and against particular treatments as well as their assessment of the needs of patients, and the juries then give their verdict. Such juries have considerable attractions in the difficult task of priority-setting, not least because they involve potential service users rather than providers. One important concern, however, is that public judgements can be more illiberal than professional ones (as in the case of capital punishment). When public assessments of different treatments were made in Oregon, a pioneer in the introduction of explicit priority-setting, services for AIDs sufferers and drug and alcohol abusers tended to be given low priority—moral worth here contributing to judgements about treatment priorities (Dixon and Welch 1991). Low priority has also been given to those with long-term problems such as those with mental illness or learning difficulties. Of course, the composition of such juries need not be restricted to lay citizens and could include clinicians and health managers, whose priorities often differ from those of the public. However, deciding on a reasonable balance is difficult, and the fact that the balance is likely to affect the outcome highlights a second, major problem with citizens' juries, which is that public priority rankings are not consistent or uniform. This is one reason why Klein and his colleagues argue that there can be no single ultimate solution to the task of priority-setting, and that what is important is to enhance the quality of decision-making, which involves 'trying to reconcile competing values, interests and concepts of the good' (Klein et al. 1996: 139).

Recent governments have tended to waver between allocating powers of priority-setting between doctors and managers. Whereas historically doctors have been the crucial priority-setters in the NHS, during the 1980s managers were given rather more power. The Labour Government's strategy is to put greater power into the hands of primary care group commissioners, including GPs, nurses, managers, and lay representatives. This has created anxieties amongst GPs that they will be held responsible for limiting access to NHS resources, and others have argued that clinicians will have too much power.[30] Whilst the primary care groups could act like the citizens' juries, reviewing the evidence and coming to their own conclusions, they need, for the reasons I have indicated, to operate within national guidelines. The advantage of primary care groups rather than hospital doctors making decisions is that they probably have a better idea of the health problems of the population as a whole and may be less wedded to expensive, high-technology solutions; however, they are more subject to pressure from patients—a further justification for national guidelines.

Conclusion

It is not easy to provide solutions to the difficult task of setting resource allocation priorities at the individual level. I have suggested that three criteria need to be taken into account: health need, health benefit, and cost. Of the three the most difficult to measure is health benefit, and given the pressures of clinicians to provide treatments it is essential that the health benefits of specific treatments are assessed very carefully, especially in relation to the precise clinical indications for their use. To achieve this scrutiny there is a need for combined national and local level assessment and regulation of treatments and health care activities. At the national level, bodies such as the National Institute for Clinical Excellence have a key role to play in ensuring adequate assessments and in establishing guidelines and protocols on treatment use.

Of course such strategies raise problems. On the one hand, they will generate opposition from the medical profession who will be likely, rightly, to see national guidelines as undermining their clinical autonomy but this is something they will have to accept. On the other hand, national guidelines may generate opposition from the public anxious that they are being denied treatments that are of potential value to them. This is where openness and public debate is so essential. And it needs to be remembered that such anxieties may well be less than the anxieties and suffering generated by the uncertainties and apparent arbitrariness of the rationing that is already occurring within the NHS.

The determining of resource allocation priorities has to be set in the context of the way in which medical care is shaped not just by health needs but by a range of external pressures, including medical and other health care professionals' own interests, the interests of pharmaceutical and other commercial companies, the media, and patient groups, all of whom exert a powerful influence on the character of health care. The determining of priorities also has to be set in the context of the way in which the health of the population is itself is shaped by a range of societal forces, forces that I examined in some detail in earlier chapters and whose role has recently been reiterated in a number of key publications (Secretary of State for Health 1998a; Acheson 1998). Whilst the aspiration that a healthier population might lead to a reduced demand for health care is almost certainly a chimera, this is not a decisive argument against a greater concentration on public health issues, including the need for important social changes, which have an intrinsic value even if they do not reduce demands on the health services. In this respect a key action that could be taken by government would be to introduce a health audit of new policies and initiatives to determine their consequences for the health of the nation. This might seem a difficult and demanding task, yet routine consideration of the health consequences of different policies is surely desirable. Such considerations already occasionally feature in public policy decisions, as when higher taxes on cigarettes and petrol are justified on health grounds. Yet attention to health in most public policy areas is currently the exception rather than the rule. Desirable though it is, the importance of clinical audit almost certainly pales into insignificance in comparison with the potential value of a routine health audit of government policy. What is needed is not so much that individuals should try to lead healthier lives but that governments and other groups should seek to ensure that their policies do not have adverse consequences for health.

Notes

Notes to Chapter 1

1 The World Health Organization's now classic definition of health is a 'state of complete physical, mental, and social well-being and not merely the absence of disease or infirmity'.

2 The Government is now planning to make a distinction between the health and social care costs of long-term care.

3 Using percentage of GDP, however, makes the differences in spending between countries look smaller than if we take absolute spending per capita. In 1991, per capita spending on health was $2,763 in the US, but only $1,039 in the UK—it was $1,869 in France and $1,588 in Germany—the GDP comparison was 12.7 per cent for the US and 6.1 per cent for the UK (Allsop 1995: 345)

4 Life expectancy is calculated by applying the death rates of a given year or set of years to a generation of say, 100,000 births, and observing their survival in the form of a life table.

5 These are life expectancy rates calculated on the basis of mortality rates in a given period—so-called 'period life expectancy'. It is also possible to calculate life expectancy for a given cohort, such as those born in a particular year—cohort life expectancy (Charlton 1997). However, for recent cohorts this involves making considerable assumptions about the mortality to which the cohort will be subject in future years.

6 The incidence of an illness refers to the number of new cases in a given period, often a year, prevalence to the number of cases at a specific time and so is affected by the duration of an illness.

7 The analogy is with the demographic transition to which it is held to be related.

8 The World Health Organization distinguishes between impairments, which are abnormalities of body structure and appearance or of organ or system function, and disabilities which represent the consequence of impairment in terms of functional performance and activity by the individual.

9 One thesis is that there is a 'compression of morbidity', with people staying active and healthier for longer and morbidity compressed into a relatively shorter period before death (Fries 1980; 1989).

10 The figure for England and Wales was down to 6 in 1996 (see Table 1.2).

11 The earlier report, *The Health of the Nation*, published by the Conservative Government did not include any international data, so that there was no indication of how Britain was doing in comparison with other countries.

12 It has to be recognized that each country has distinctive patterns of ill-health and that high levels of heart disease in Britain are matched by high levels of

alcohol-related problems in France, and high levels of cancer in Scandinavia (Wilkinson 1996: 62).

13 It is more of a problem in developing countries than in Britain, though there is a growing concern in Britain about TB in cattle.

14 In the eighteenth century gin-drinking was a major social problem, but it was not treated as a problem of mental health (Porter 1990).

15 The identification of deaths as due to suicide is a complex social process where cultural beliefs and values play an important role. But such factors are unlikely to account for the changes over the last three decades in death rates from suicides.

16 *Our Healthier Nation* gives less attention to these factors than the earlier *Health of the Nation* report. Instead, and rightly in my view, it focuses far more on the social and environmental causes of illness.

17 The Conservative Government's *The Health of the Nation* set targets for four areas of risk: smoking, diet and nutrition, blood pressure, and sexual health.

18 For a helpful discussion of recent debates on social class, see Annandale (1997: ch. 4).

19 Though these data are all based on the Registrar-General's social-class classification, there have been some changes over time in the way in which occupations have been classified.

20 Illsley and Le Grand (1987) argue that changes in the class composition of the population make occupation an unsatisfactory measure of temporal changes in inequalities in health. They contend that regional differences in health provide a better measure of temporal changes in socio-economic inequalities in health, and that these show a reduction in inequalities over the period since 1931, especially in the younger age groups (Illsley et al. 1991).

21 The most recent data indicate that income inequalities have stabilized over the last few years.

22 Male deaths from coronary heart disease have declined particularly in the middle classes.

Notes to Chapter 2

1 This point is discussed further in Chapter 3.

2 Data on sun-burning is now included in *Social Trends*, (ONS 1999: Chapter 7).

3 It is important to remember that taking risks may itself bring excitement and pleasure.

4 The term 'clinical' means 'of or at the sick-bed'.

5 Data from the Netherlands and Denmark do not support the Health and Lifestyle Survey finding that unhealthy behaviour is of little importance to those in unfavourable circumstances, the authors concluding that this is probably because the disadvantaged groups in these two countries are better off than those in a similar position in Britain (Kooiker and Christansen 1995).

6 Geographical location is equally important in the case of fallout from the

Chernobyl disaster where, as I have argued, it would also be inappropriate to think in terms of individual behaviour

7 The best known of these is the Holmes-Rahe (1967) Social Readjustment Rating Scale.

8 Brown and Harris's (1978) is the best known of the measures that make some external assessment of the significance of the event/circumstance to the individual.

9 The study focused on women: it was easier to obtain a sample of depressed women, as depression is more commonly identified in women than in men. The salient vulnerability factors would not be identical in men, and also vary across time and place.

10 There is already debate about whether its powers will be sufficiently extensive.

11 For Marx, alienation was objective rather than subjective, and characterized the worker's objective relation to what was produced.

12 In earlier papers he has emphasized the role of material factors in accounting for class inequalities in health. See Wilkinson (1986b).

13 Recent figures on the growth of single-parent families are provided in Chapter 3.

Notes to Chapter 3

1 Ethnic inequalities are not examined in this chapter for reasons of space. Nazroo (1997a) argues they can largely be accounted for by class but this is a contested issue (see Chapter 1).

2 The concept of case-fatality provides a useful way of measuring the outcome of illness, an outcome that may or may not be affected positively or negatively by medical intervention.

3 The period 1870–96 is usually termed 'the great depression'.

4 A comparison of male and female death rates classified by husband's occupation has sometimes been used as a basis for making a prima facie case as to whether or not mortality levels are being affected by occupation-related mortality. Where husbands' and wives' death rates diverge considerably, occupation related factors may be at work; where they coincide, it may be less the occupation per se that is important than the standard of living associated with it (see e.g. Benjamin 1968: 93).

5 In this respect the effect of the world-wide depression was partly paid by Britain's colonial empire—countries which were an important source of imported foods and were forced to lower their prices.

6 Jane Austen, born in 1777, whose father was a clergyman, had five brothers, one of whom was disabled and did not marry. The first wives of three of her brothers died after childbirth, two after their eleventh child was born, both before the age of 40, the other after her fourth child before she was 25; the fourth wife who had one child by her first marriage died aged 51 of cancer. This picture was not untypical (Tomalin 1997).

7 Not having a paid job is nowadays negatively associated with health for women,

even allowing for the effects of selection according to health status. However, the cost and benefits of non-participation depend on employment conditions and a number of other factors such as community networks, so that we cannot simply apply findings from the 1980s and 1990s to the 1920s and 1930s.

8 Stays in TB sanitoria were also included—significant at a time when TB was a important source of mortality.

9 The height requirement was reduced in the First World War. This means that in fact health had improved between the two wars (Blane 1987).

10 There was nonetheless considerable reluctance to accept the link between poverty and nutrition.

11 Wilkinson also includes a lengthy discussion of the importance of relative over absolute poverty, though as he notes this can only be studied by comparing societies, since at an individual level the two cannot be measured independently.

12 Wilkinson suggests, incorrectly, that there was no rationing during the First World War, though it was certainly far more limited.

13 The major developments of penicillin occurred during the war, which probably encouraged rather than reduced scientific innovation in medicine (as elsewhere).

14 The fact that longevity is on average higher in women than in men might seem to call into question this emphasis on the importance of poverty to health, since poverty is more common amongst women than men. However, poverty can still be important in accounting for class differences in health between women or between men. Moreover, it is worth noting that female life expectancy in women is lower in Britain than in other European countries (whereas male life expectancy is amongst the highest in Europe), and it may well be poverty (which is greater in Britain than in many other European countries) that is having an adverse effect on women's mortality.

15 Having three children under 14 at home was one of Brown and Harris's vulnerability factors for depression in women (1978).

Notes to Chapter 4

1 Aneurin Bevan (Foot 1975) argued that the inclusion of mental health services was important because of the linkage between mental and physical illness.

2 The models are constructed around medical care because the employment status of doctors is one factor differentiating the models, but for the most part the terms 'medical care' and 'health care' can be used interchangeably.

3 The controversial use of the Private Finance Initiative as a means of getting private companies to build hospitals, in effect leased to the NHS, will mean that some NHS hospitals are not publicly owned, though they will continue to be publicly managed and controlled.

4 The insured had to register with a 'panel' doctor, one who had been approved for inclusion in the scheme, and was put on the panel (list).

5 GPs argued that a salaried practice would interfere with their clinical freedom. One of the changes introduced was that GPs were no longer allowed to sell their practice as a business.

6 NHS dentists have typically been paid for work with children on a capitation basis.

7 A very recent development had been the growth of private drop-in surgeries in locations such as major rail stations in London. The company Boots is now setting up private dental services in a few of its shops.

8 A clear example of this was when the Conservative conference at the Grand Hotel in Brighton was disrupted by a bomb, and the injured politicians became emergency patients at NHS hospitals, notwithstanding the fact that many would have had private medical insurance.

9 In 1980 the government introduced tax concessions to employers taking out insurance for workers paid less than £8,500; in 1990 tax concessions on private medical insurance were introduced for the elderly; they have been withdrawn by the Labour Government.

10 Marginally fewer women than men tend to be covered, mainly because of the provision of private medical insurance as an employment benefit which, given occupational differences, is far more common for men than women, though wives and children are often covered by their husbands' insurance.

11 The figures for England are published in the Department of Health's annual *Health and Personal Social Services for England*. For Wales, Scotland, and Northern Ireland they are available from the respective Departments/Offices.

12 The figures supplied by the respective Departments/Offices are: England 193,625 beds, Scotland 37,998, Wales 15,194, and Northern Ireland 9,006.

13 The Act introduced a key distinction between purchasers and providers, the main purchasers being the health authorities and GP fundholders (GP practices that met certain criteria, mainly size), and the main providers being the new hospital and other trusts as well as GPs.

14 Under the Conservatives the phrase was 'primary care-led NHS'.

15 The characteristics of biomedicine are outlined in a number of places (see e.g. Mishler and AmaraSingham, 1991).

16 An obvious example is the failure to test new treatments adequately; see Chapter 6.

17 Drugs are widely used in hospices to relieve pain.

18 The obvious exception is AIDs, an infectious disease which generated major concerns, but the health campaigns mainly focused on health promotion.

19 Public health work as defined here raises fewer questions about individual control and surveillance, though there are still very significant ethical issues.

20 The current government standard is that no patient should have to wait more than 18 months for an operation, though this is not always achieved.

21 There can be indirect financial incentives, as when a higher salary follows the

public recognition and prestige arising from certain types of medical innovation.

Notes to Chapter 5

1 Clearly ideas about medicine and nursing as 'vocations' are underpinned by such beliefs.

2 Role analysis was criticized in the 1950s and 1960s, and the term 'role' is not now a widely used sociological concept. However, we can talk instead of tasks and duties.

3 Its significance for the family and the wider society differs.

4 In some societies young children are an important source of labour both within and outside the family.

5 Significantly employers have been markedly reluctant to invest in health care themselves even though the loss of skilled workers can be costly.

6 A criticism also often made of Marxist accounts that are functionalist in character.

7 In this respect Parsons's point about the isolation of the sick from each other needs to be modified, particularly where sickness is chronic.

8 Jane Becker, a Ph.D. student in the Department of Sociology at the University of Essex, is currently researching the role and activities of these clinics.

9 One of the disadvantages of private insurance is that that those with certain known health problems may not be able to find any company willing to give them insurance, and if they do premiums may be higher. Premiums are usually also age-related, so that the elderly face the highest premiums at the point in the lifecycle when their income usually declines and their health may start to deteriorate.

10 Ian Gough (1979) offers a similar analysis of the development of welfare states, arguing that two factors—class struggle and 'the ability of the capitalist state to secure the long-term reproduction of class relations'—were crucial.

11 The 3rd edition of the book (1995) divides the period from the 1980s onwards into several phases, but I find this framework less helpful.

12 The estimate of £176 million was derived from an appendix to the Beveridge report which had costed the service at £170 million per annum, although Beveridge had not provided a detailed financial plan. The NHS Bill of 1946 had costed the service at £152 million per annum.

Notes to Chapter 6

1 Predictably, there are debates about how far the extra £21 million over 3 years announced by the Government in 1998 represents a real increase in funding to the NHS.

2 Klein et al. list 7 forms of rationing: by denial (which I have called exclusion), by selection, by deflection, by deterrence, by delay, by dilution, and by termination (1996: 11–12).

3 Klein et al. see these individual-level decisions as the ones where the term rationing 'in its strict sense' is appropriate (1996: 10).

4 The case for making these priority areas was based on the comparatively low levels of NHS spending, and the recognition of service inadequacies. They were to be made priorities precisely because they had not been.

5 This is not to say that mobility is fully restored.

6 This definition could equally apply to the term 'illness', but I have used the term 'health problem' because it suggests a greater breadth.

7 This is the estimate given in a paper by the Nuffield Institute for Health Care (1996).

8 There was recent concern when one type of prosthesis was found to wear out very quickly, resulting in the need for these prostheses to be replaced at considerable expense. Significantly, the most reliable prostheses are by no means the most expensive (Nuffield Institute for Health Care 1996).

9 Younger people with severe hip problems may well have a higher chance of a hip replacement than, say, a person over 80 with the same level of problem.

10 The effectiveness of an intervention is a matter of whether it achieves its objectives and how well it does so, which involves some comparison either with those not receiving any treatment at all or with those receiving some alternative treatment.

11 It is important to note that not all medical interventions need to be subject to systematic evaluation. Some procedures such as bone-setting can be adequately evaluated without the need for double-blind trials.

12 There is some systematic evaluation of the performance of different prostheses.

13 There is some consideration of the link between diets, exercise, and osteoporosis.

14 This is not a requirement for the licensing of treatments in the UK.

15 The Royal College of Psychiatrist's recent work and publicity on 'undetected' depression in men has been funded by the drug companies.

16 There is some evidence of somewhat higher levels of depression than formerly, though this may partly arise from a changing consciousness of depression in men and in part from changing boundaries.

17 The first list was very restrictive and has recently been expanded.

18 Psychiatry is one area where such drug cocktails are not uncommon. A patient might be on one or even two anti-psychotic drugs, one or two drugs to try to counter some of their side-effects, some form of sleeping tablet, and a drug for a physical problem.

19 This point was captured forcefully and polemically by Ivan Illich, who asserted that professionals 'gain legal power to create the need that, by law, they alone will be allowed to satisfy' (1977: 16).

20 Scheff argued that the stigma and its associated adverse effects arising from being labelled mentally ill were very considerable.

21 This point has been established in range of studies. For instance, Blum (1978)

analysed admissions data from a New Haven psychiatric hospital and showed a shift away from diagnoses of anxiety neurosis, which Freudian ideas had made fashionable, towards diagnoses of depression with the development of new anti-depressants in the 20 years between the mid-1950s and the mid-1970s.

22 Preliminary tests have to be carried out on healthy individuals.

23 Although attractive in their simplicity, these new measures have drawbacks in the assumption they make that cases are equivalent and can be simply added together. They tend to draw attention away from consideration of the specific clinical indications for the use of particular treatments.

24 These are already published in Scotland.

25 This standard has already been criticized by some doctors who argue that not all cancers progress rapidly; however, the government's concern is to provide general reassurance about access to treatment, and introducing qualifications would undermine the power of its message.

26 Twenty-one per cent of health authorities responding to a survey in 1992 indicated that they had made some use of QALYs in priority setting (Robinson and New 1992).

27 A local psychiatrist (personal communication) recently commented that 'the jury is out' on Clozapine, and said that one problem was that if the drug were stopped symptoms tended to return with particular force.

28 It is important to note that possible long-term savings are often invoked to justify high short-term expenditure on treatment, but frequently this is a form of polemic which is not grounded in a careful cost–benefit analysis.

29 The construction of eligibility criteria constitutes an explicit rationing device that proceeds with recognition of the limited availability of some form of treatment or care and then constructs criteria as to who should receive the limited resources. It differs from work on clinical protocols which starts not from the premise of limited resources but from the premise of trying to determine the boundaries of the value of particular treatments and from the assumption that the value of a treatment will vary significantly for different patient groups.

30 GPs are to chair the primary care groups and will be in the majority.

References

Abel-Smith, B. (1964), *The Hospitals, 1800–1948*, London: Heinemann.

—— (1994), *An Introduction to Health: Policy, Planning and Financing*, London: Longman.

Abraham, J. (1995), *Science, Politics and the Pharmaceutical Industry: Controversy and Bias in Drug Regulation*, London: UCL Press.

Acheson, D. (1998), *Independent Inquiry into Inequalities in Health Report*. London: Stationery Office.

Allsop, J. (1995), *Health Policy and the NHS: Towards 2000*, 2nd edn, London: Longman.

Andrews, A., and Jewson, N. (1993), 'Ethnicity and Infant Deaths: The Implications of Recent Statistical Evidence for Materialist Explanations', *Sociology of Health and Illness*, 15: 137–56.

Annandale, E. (1997), *Sociology of Health and Medicine*, Cambridge: Polity.

Antonovosky, A. (1989), 'Social Inequalities in Health: A Complementary Perspective', in J. Fox (ed.), *Health Inequalities in European Countries*, Aldershot: Gower.

Arber, S. (1989), 'Gender and Class Inequalities in Health: Understanding the Differentials', in J. Fox (ed.), *Health Inequalities in European Countries*, Aldershot: Gower.

—— and Ginn, J. (1991), *Gender and Later Life: A Sociological Analysis of Resources and Constraints*, London: Sage.

Armstrong, D. (1995), 'The Rise of Surveillance Medicine', *Sociology of Health and Illness*, 17: 393–404.

Audit Commission (1994), *Finding a Place: A Review of Mental Health Services for Adults*, London: HMSO.

Barrett, M., and McIntosh, M. (1980), 'The "Family Wage": Some Problems for Socialists and Feminists', *Capital and Class*, 11: 51–72.

Bartley, M. (1993), 'Health and labour force participation: "stress", selection and the reproduction costs of labour power', *Journal of Social Policy*, 20: 327–64.

—— Lynch, K., Sacker, A., and Dodgeon, B. (1998), 'Social Variations in Health: Relationship of Mortality to the ONS Socio-Economic Class (SEC) Schema', paper given to the SEC Validation Workshop, University of Essex, Dec. 1998.

—— Popay, J., and Plewis, I. (1992), 'Domestic Conditions, Paid Employment and Women's Experience of Ill-health', *Sociology of Health and Illness*, 14: 313–43.

Bartrip, P. (1985), 'The Rise and Decline of Workmen's Compensation', in P. Weindling (ed.), *The Social History of Occupational Health*, London: Croom Helm.

Benjamin, B. (1968), *Demographic Analysis*. London: Allen and Unwin.

Benzeval, M., Judge, K., and Whitehead, M. (eds.) (1995), *Tackling Inequalities in Health: An Agenda for Action*. London: King's Fund.

Bernstein, W. (1955), *Regulating Business by Independent Commission*. Princeton: Princeton University Press.

Beveridge, W. (1942) *Social Insurance and Allied Services*. London: HMSO.

Blane, D. (1987), 'The Value of Labour-Power and Health', in G. Scambler (ed.), *Sociological Theory and Medical Sociology*, London: Tavistock.

—— Davey Smith, G., and Bartley, M. (1993), 'Social Selection: What Does It Contribute to Social Class Differences in Health?' *Sociology of Health and Illness*, 15: 1–15.

—— Montgomery, S. M., and Berney, D. R. (1998), 'Research Note: Social Class Differences in Lifetime Exposure to Environmental Hazards', *Sociology of Health and Illness*, 20: 532–6.

Blauner, R. (1964), *Alienation and Freedom*, Chicago: Chicago University Press.

Blaxter, M. (1990), *Health and Lifestyles*, London: Routledge.

Blum, J, (1978), 'On Changes in Psychiatric Diagnosis over Time', *American Psychologist*, 33: 1017–31.

Bordo, S. (1990), 'Reading the Slender Body', in M. Jacobus, E. F. Keller, and S. Shuttleworth (eds.), *Body/Politics: Women and the Discourse of Science*, London: Routledge.

Bosma, H., Marmot, M. G., Hemingway, H., Nicholson, A. C., Brunner, E., and Stansfield, S. A. (1997), 'Low Job Control and Risk of Coronary Heart Disease in Whitehall II (Prospective Cohort Study)', *British Medical Journal*, 314: 558–65.

Bowling, A. (1987), 'Mortality after Bereavement: A Review of the Literature on Survival Periods and Factors Affecting Survival', *Social Science and Medicine*, 24: 117–24.

Brenner, H. (1973), *Mental Illness and the Economy*, Cambridge, Mass.: Harvard University Press.

Brown, G. and Harris, T. (1978), *Social Origins of Depression*, London: Tavistock.

—— —— (1989), *Life Events and Illness*, London: Unwin Hyman.

Brugha, T. S. (1995), 'Social Support and Psychiatric Disorder: Overview of Evidence', in T. S. Brugha (ed.) *Social Support and Psychiatric Disorder*, Cambridge: Cambridge University Press.

Bryder, L. (1988), *Below the Magic Mountain: A Social History of Tuberculosis in Twentieth-Century Britain*, Oxford: Clarendon Press.

Bunting, J. (1997), 'Morbidity and Health-related Behaviour of Adults: A Review', in F. Drever and M. Whitehead (eds.), *Health Inequalities*, London: Stationery Office.

Burnett, J. (1968), *Plenty and Want: A Social History of Diet in England from 1815 to the Present Day*, Harmondsworth: Penguin.

Busfield, J. (1986), *Managing Madness: Changing Ideas and Practice*. London: Hutchinson.

—— (1990), 'Sectoral Divisions in Consumption: The Case of Medical Care', *Sociology*, 24: 77–96.

—— (1996), *Men, Women and Madness: Understanding Gender and Mental Disorder*. London: Macmillan.

—— and Paddon, M. (1977), *Thinking about Children: Sociology and Fertility in Post-War England*, Cambridge: Cambridge University Press.

Calder, A. (1969), *The People's War*, London: Jonathan Cape.

Caselli, G. and Lopez, A. D. (eds.) (1996), *Health and Mortality among Elderly Populations*, Oxford: Clarendon Press.

Central Statistical Office (CSO) (1971), *Social Trends* 1, London: HMSO.

—— (1985), *Annual Abstract of Statistics 1985*, London: HMSO.

Chadwick, E. (1965) [1842], *Report on the Sanitary Condition of the Labouring Population of Great Britain*, Edinburgh: University Press.

Charlton, J. (1997), 'Trends in All-cause Mortality, 1841–1994', in Office for National Statistics, *The Health of Adult Britain, 1841–1994*, i. London: Stationery Office.

Clare, A. (1980), *Psychiatry in Dissent*, 2nd edn. London: Tavistock.

Cobb, S., and Kasl, S. V. (1977), *Termination: The Consequences of Job Loss*, DHEW-NIOSH Publication no. 77-224. Cincinnati: National Institute for Ocupational Health and Safety.

Cochrane, A. L. (1972), *Effectiveness and Efficiency: Random Reflections on Health Services*, London: Nuffield Provincial Hospitals Trust.

Collins, E., and Klein, R. (1980), 'Equity and the NHS: Self-reported Morbidity, Access and Primary Care'. *British Medical Journal*, 251: 1111–15.

Constantine, S. (1977), *Social Conditions in Britain between the Wars*. Harmondsworth: Penguin.

Cooper, C. L., Fargher, E. B., Bray, C. L., and Ramsdale, D. R. (1985), 'The Significance of Psychosocial Factors in Predicting Coronary Heart Disease in Patients with Valvular Heart Disease', *Social Science and Medicine*, 20: 315–18.

Cooper L. (1998), 'Contested Knowledge, Constructed Illness? The ME Controversy', PhD. thesis, Department of Sociology, University of Essex.

Coreil, J., Levin, J. S., and Jaco, G. (1994), *Health and Social Change in International Perspective*, Boston: Harvard School of Public Health.

Coulter, A. (1992), 'The Interface between Primary and Secondary Care', in M. Roland and A. Coulter (eds.), *Hospital Referrals*. Oxford: Oxford University Press.

David, E. (1977), *English Bread and Yeast Cookery*. London: Allen Lane.

Davies, C. (1995), *Gender and the Professional Predicament in Nursing*, Buckingham: Open University Press.

Davis, P. (1997), *Managing Medicines: Public Policy and Therapeutic Drugs*, Buckingham: Open University Press.

Department of Health (DOH) (1996), *Hospital Episode Statistics*. London: Stationery Office.

Department of Health and Social Security (DHSS) (1976), *Priorities for Health and Personal Social Services: A Consultative Document*, London: HMSO.

—— (1983), *Report of the NHS Management Inquiry* (the Griffiths Report). London: DHSS.

—— (1986) *Report of the Committee of Enquiry into Unnecessary Dental Treatment*, London: HMSO.

Department of Social Security (1997), *Family Resources Survey*, London: Stationery Office.

Dixon, J., and Welch, H. G. (1991), 'Priority Setting: Lessons from Oregon', *The Lancet*, 337, 13 Apr. 891–4.

Donnison, J. (1977), *Midwives and Medical Men: A History of Inter-Professional Rivalries and Women's Rights*, London: Heinemann.

Doyal, L., and Gough, I. (1991). *A Theory of Human Need*. London: Macmillan.

Drever, F., and Whitehead, M. (1997), *Health Inequalities*, Office for National Statistics, London: Stationery Office.

Dubos, R. (1968), *Man, Medicine, and Environment*, Harmondsworth: Penguin.

Durkheim, E. (1964) [1893], *The Division of Labour in Society*, New York: Free Press.

Eckstein, H. (1958), *The English Health Service: Its Origins, Structure and Achievements*, Cambridge, Mass.: Harvard University Press.

Elstad, J. I. (1996), 'How Large Are the Differences Really? Self-reported Long-standing Illness among Working Class and Middle Class Men', *Sociology of Health and Illness*, 18: 475–98.

—— (1998), 'Psycho-Social Perspectives on Social Inequalities in Health', *Sociology of Health and Illness*, 20: 598–618.

Esping-Andersen, G. (1990), *The Three Worlds of Welfare Capitalism*, Cambridge: Polity.

Ettorre, E., and Riska, E. (1995), *Gendered Moods: Psychotropics and Society*, London: Routledge.

Farrow, S. and Jewell, D. (1993), 'Opening the Gate: Referrals from Primary to Secondary Care', in S. Frankel and R. West (eds.), *Rationing and Rationality in the National Health Service*, London: Macmillan.

Finch, J. (1983), *Married to the Job*. London: Allen and Unwin.

Foot, M. (1975), *Aneurin Bevan 1945–1960*, St Albans: Paladin.

Foucault, M. (1973), *The Birth of the Clinic: An Archaeology of Medical Perception*. London: Tavistock.

—— (1991), 'On Governmentality', in G. Burchell, C. Gordon, and P. Miller (eds.), *The Foucault Effect: Studies in Governmentality*, London: Harvester Wheatsheaf.

Fox, J., Goldblatt, P., and Jones, D. (1990), 'Social Class Mortality Differentials: Artefact, Selection or Life Circumstances?', in J. Goldblatt (ed.), *Longitudinal Study: Mortality and Social Organisation, 1970–1981*, OPCS Series LS no. 6, London: HMSO.

Fox J. and Benzeval, M. (1995), 'Perspectives on Social Variations in Health', in M. Benzeval, K. Judge and M. Whitehead (eds), *Tackling Inequalities in Health*, London: Kings Fund.

Freidson, E. (1970), *Profession of Medicine*, New York: Dodd, Mead.

—— (1994), *Professionalism Reborn*, Cambridge: Polity.

Frenk, J., Bobadilla, J.-L., Stern, C., Frejka, T., and Lozano, R. (1991), 'Elements for a Theory of the Health Transition', *Health Transition Review*, 1: 21–38.

Fries, J. F. (1980), 'Ageing, Natural Death and the Compression of Morbidity', *New England Journal of Medicine*, 3030: 130–5.

—— (1989), 'Reduction of the National Morbidity', in S. Lewis (ed.), *Aging and Health*, Mich.: Lewis.

Gabe, J., Kelleher, D. and Williams, G. (eds) (1994), *Challenging Medicine*, London: Routledge.

Galbraith, S. and McCormick, A. (1997), 'Infection in England and Wales, 1838–1993', in Office for National Statistics, *The Health of Adult Britain, 1841–1994*, ii. London: Stationery Office.

Gerhardt, U. (1989), *Ideas about Illness: An Intellectual and Political History of Medical Sociology*, London: Macmillan.

Giddens, A. (1991), *Modernity and Self-Identity: Self and Society in the Late Modern Age*. Cambridge: Polity.

Gough, I. (1979), *The Political Economy of the Welfare State*, London: Macmillan.

Graham, H. (1985), 'Providers, Negotiators and Mediators: Women as the Hidden Carers', in E. Lewin and V. Olesen (eds.), *Women, Health and Healing*, London: Tavistock.

—— (1987), 'Women's Smoking and Family Health', *Social Science and Medicine*, 25: 47–56.

—— and Blackburn, C. (1998), 'Socio-economic Patterning of Health and Smoking Behaviour among Mothers with Children on Income Support', *Sociology of Health and Illness*, 20: 215–40.

Griffith, B. and Rayner, G., (1985), *Commercial Medicine in London*, London: Greater London Council.

Harrison, G., Owens, D., Holton, A., Neilson, D., and Boot, D. (1988), 'A Prospective Study of Severe Mental Disorder in Afro-Caribbean Patients', *Psychological Medicine*, 18: 643–57.

Hart, N, (1989), 'Sex, Gender and Survival: Inequalities of Life Chances between European Men and Women', in J. Fox (ed.), *Health Inequalities in European Countries*, Aldershot: Gower.

Hattersley, L. (1997) 'Expectation of Life by Social Class', in F. Drever and M. Whitehead (eds.), *Health Inequalities*, London: Stationery Office.

Health Education Authority (1994), *Black and Minority Ethnic Groups in England*. London: Health Education Authority.

—— (1996), *Health in England 1995*. London: Stationery Office.

Higgins, J. (1988), *The Business of Medicine: Private Health Care in Britain*, London: Macmillan.

Hobsbawm, E. J. (1969), *Industry and Empire*, Harmondsworth: Penguin,

Holmes, T. H. and Rahe, R. M. (1967), 'The Social Re-adjustment Rating Scale', *Journal of Psychosomatic Research*, 11: 213–18.

Hopkins, E. (1979), *A Social History of the English Working Classes, 1815–1945*, London: Edward Arnold.

Horwitz, A. (1977), 'The Pathways into Psychiatric Treatment: Some Differences between Men and Women', *Journal of Health and Social Behaviour*, 18: 169–78.

Howell, J. D. (1995), *Technology in the Hospital: Transforming Patient Care in the Early Twentieth Century*. Baltimore: Johns Hopkins University Press.

Hunter, D.J. (19994), 'From Tribalism to Corporatism: The Managerial Challenge to Medical Dominance', in J. Gabe, D. Kelleher, and G. Williams (eds.), *Challenging Medicine*. London: Routledge.

Illich, I. (1977) 'Disabling Professions', in I. Illich, I. K. Zola, J. McKnight, J. Caplan, and H. Shaiken, *Disabling Professions*, London: Marion Boyars.

Illsley, R., and Le Grand, J. (1987), 'The Measurement of Inequality in Health', in A. Williams (ed.), *Economics and Health*, London: Macmillan.

—— —— and Mullings, J. (1991), *Regional Inequalities in Mortality*, Discussion Paper WHP/57, London: Suntory–Toyota International Centre for Economics and Related Disciplines.

James, O. (1997), *Britain on the Couch*. London: Century.

Jewson, N. D. (1976), 'The Disappearance of the Sick-man from Medical Cosmology', *Sociology* 10: 225–44.

Johansson, S. R. (1991), 'The Health Transition: The Cultural Inflation of Morbidity during the Decline of Mortality', *Health Transition Review*, 1: 39–68.

Johnson, T. J. (1972), *Professions and Power*, London: Macmillan.

—— (1995), 'Governmentality and the Institutionalization of Expertise', in T. Johnson, G. Larkin, and M. Saks (eds.), *Health Professions and the State in Europe*, London: Routledge.

Judge, K., Mulligan, J., and Benzeval, M. (1998), 'Income Inequality and Population Health', *Social Science and Medicine*, 46: 567–79.

Kendell, R. (1975), 'The Concept of Disease and Its Implications for Psychiatry', *British Journal of Psychiatry*, 117: 305–15.

King, L.S. (1954), 'What Is Disease?' *Philosophy of Science*, 21: 193–203.

Klein, R. (1989), *The Politics of the National Health Service*, 2nd edn, London: Longman.

—— (1995), *The New Politics of the National Health Service*, 3rd edn, London: Longman.

—— Day, P., and Remayne, S. (1996), *Priority Setting and Rationing in the National Health Service*. Buckingham: Open University Press.

Kleinman, A. (1987), 'Anthropology and Psychiatry: The Role of Culture in Cross-cultural Research on Illness', *British Journal of Psychiatry*, 151: 447–54.

—— (1988), *The Illness Narratives: Suffering, Healing and the Human Condition*. New York: Basic Books.

Kooiker, S., and Christiansen, T. (1995), 'Inequalities in Health: The Interaction of Circumstances and Health Related Behaviour', *Sociology of Health and Illness*, 17: 495–524.

Kramer, P. (1994), *Listening to Prozac*, London: Fourth Estate.

Kuhn, A., and Wolpe, A. M. (1978), *Feminism and Materialism*, London: Routledge and Kegan Paul.

Laing, R. D. (1960), *The Divided Self*, London: Tavistock.

—— (1967), *The Politics of Experience and the Bird of Paradise*, Harmondsworth: Penguin.

Larson, M. (1977), *The Rise of Professionalism*, California: University of California Press.

Lasch, C. (1979), *Haven in a Heartless World*, New York: Basic Books.

Le Grand, J. (1982), *The Strategy of Equality*, London: Allen and Unwin.

Lewis, J. (1980), *The Politics of Motherhood: Child and Maternal Welfare in England, 1900–1939*. London: Croom Helm.

—— (1983), 'Dealing with Dependency: State Practices and Social Realities, 1870–1945', in J. Lewis (ed.), *Women's Welfare: Women's Rights*, London: Croom Helm.

—— (1986), *What Price Community Medicine*? Brighton: Wheatsheaf.

Light, D. (1995), 'Countervailing Powers: A Framework for the Professions in Transition', in T. Johnson, G. Larkin, and M. Saks (eds.), *Health Professions and the State in Europe*, London: Routledge.

Lindsey, A. (1962), *Socialized Medicine in England and Wales: The National Health Service, 1948–1961*, Chapel Hill: University of North Carolina Press.

Macdonald, K. (1995), *The Sociology of the Professions*. London: Sage.

MacDonald, M. (1981), *Mystical Bedlam: Madness, Anxiety and Healing in Seventeenth-Century England*, Cambridge: Cambridge University Press.

Macfarlane, A. (1990), 'Official Statistics and Women's Health', in H. Roberts (ed.), *Women's Health Counts*, London: Routledge.

MacIntyre, S. (1993), 'Gender Differences in the Perception of Common Cold Symptoms', *Social Science and Medicine*, 36: 15–20.

McKeown, T. (1976) *The Modern Rise of Population*, London: Edward Arnold.

McKinley, J. B. (1977), 'The Business of Good Doctoring or Doctoring as good Business: Reflections on Freidson's View of the Medical Game', *International Journal of Health Services*, 7: 459–83.

Manton, K. G. (1982), 'Changing Concepts of Morbidity and Mortality in the Elderly Population', *Milbank Memorial Fund Quarterly*, 60: 183–244.

Marinker, M. (1990), 'Principles', in M. Marinker (ed.), *Medical Audit and General Practice*. London: MSD Foundation.

Marks, G., and Barney P. (1997), 'Diseases of the Respiratory System', in Office for National Statistics, *The Health of Adult Britain 1841–1994*, ii. London: Stationery Office.

Marmot, M. G., Adelstein, A. M., Bulusu, L., and OPCS (1984), *Immigrant Mortality in England and Wales 1970–78: Causes of Death by Country of Birth*. London: HMSO.

—— Bosma, H., Hemingway, H., Brunner, E., and Stansfield, S. (1997), 'Contribution of Job Control and Other Risk Factors to Social Variations in Coronary Heart Disease Incidence', *Lancet*, 350: 235–9.

—— Rose, G., Shipley, M., and Hamilton, P. J. S (1978), 'Employment Grade and Coronary Heart Disease in British Civil Servants', *Journal of Epidemiology and Community Health*, 32: 244–9.

Martin, J., and Roberts, C. (1984), *Women and Employment: A Lifetime Perspective*, London: HMSO.

Meltzer, H., Gill, B., Pettigrew, M., and Hinds, K. (1995), *The Prevalence of Psychiatric Morbidity among Adults Living in Private Households*, London: HMSO.

Ministry of Health (1962), *Hospital Plan*, London: HMSO.

Mishler, E. G., and AmeraSingham, L. R. (1981), *Social Contexts of Health, Illness and Patient Care*, Cambridge: Cambridge University Press.

Moran. M (1994), 'Health Care Policy', in J. Clasen and R. Freeman (eds.), *Social Policy in Germany*, Hemel Hempstead: Harvester Wheatsheaf.

Muir Gray, J. A. (1997), *Evidence-Based Healthcare*, Edinburgh: Churchill Livingstone.

Mull, J., and Mull, D. (1988), 'Mothers' Concept of Childhood Diarrhoea in Rural Pakistan: What ORT Planners Should Know', *Social Science and Medicine*, 27: 53–67.

Murphy, R. (1984), 'The Structures of Closure: A Critique and Development of the Theories of Weber, Collins and Parkin', *British Journal of Sociology*, 35: 547–67.

Nathanson, C. A. (1977), 'Sex, Illness and Medical Care: A Review of Data, Theory and Methods', *Social Science and Medicine*, 11: 13.

National Audit Office (1996), *Health of the Nation: A Progress Report*, London: HMSO.

Navarro, V. (1976), *Medicine under Capitalism*, New York: Prodist.

—— (1977), 'Political Power, the State, and Their Implications in Medicine', *Review of Radical Political Economics*, 9: 61–80.

—— (1978), *Class Struggle, the State and Medicine: An Historical and Contemporary Analysis of the Medical Sector in Great Britain*, London: Martin Robertson.

Nazroo, J. Y. (1997a), *The Health of Britain's Ethnic Minorities*, London: Policy Studies Institute.

—— (1997b), *Ethnicity and Mental Health: Findings from a National Community Survey*. London: Policy Studies Institute.

Nettleton, S. (1995), *The Sociology of Health and Illness*. London: Polity.

Nuffield Institute for Health Care (1996), 'Total Hip Replacement', *Effective Health Care*, 2, 7.

Oakley, A. (1983), 'Women and Health Policy', in J. Lewis (ed.), *Women's Welfare: Women's Rights*. London: Croom Helm.

—— (1986), *The Captured Womb: A History of the Medical Care of Pregnant Women*, Oxford: Blackwell.

O'Connor, J. (1973), *The Fiscal Crisis of the State*, New York: St. Martin's Press.

Office for National Statistics (ONS) (1997a), *Annual Abstract of Statistics 1997*, London: Stationery Office.

—— (1997b), *Living in Britain 1995: General Household Survey*. London: Stationary Office.

—— (1997c), *Social Trends*, 27, London: Stationery Office.

—— (1998a), *Annual Abstract of Statistics 1997*, London: Stationery Office.

—— (1998b), *Living in Britain 1996: General Household Survey*. London: Stationery Office.

—— (1998c), *Social Trends*, 28, London: Stationery Office.

—— (1999), *Social Trends*, 29, London: Stationery Office.

Office of Population Censuses and Surveys (1978), *Mortality Statistics 1975*, Series DH1, No. 2, London: HMSO.

Omran, A.R. (1971), 'The Epidemiologic Transition: A Theory of the Epidemiology of Population Change', *Milbank Memorial Fund Quarterly*, 64: 509–38.

Padesky, C. A., and Hammen, C. L. (1981), 'Sex Differences in Depressive Symptom Expression and Help-seeking among College Students', *Sex Roles*, 7: 309–20.

Parkin, F. (1979), *Marxism and Class Theory: A Bourgeois Critique*, London: Tavistock.

Parsons, T. (1951), *The Social System*. London: Routledge and Kegan Paul.

Pelling, M. and Webster, C. (1979), 'Medical Practitioners', in C. Webster (ed.), *Health, Medicine and Mortality in the Sixteenth Century*. Cambridge: Cambridge University Press.

Phillimore, P., Beattie, A., and Townsend, P. (1994), 'The Widening Gap: Inequality of Health in Northern England, 1981–1991', *British Medical Journal*, 308: 1125–8.

Phillips, D. L., and Segal, B. F. (1969), 'Sexual Status and Psychiatric Symptoms', *American Sociological Review*, 34: 58–72.

Plant, M. A. (1997), 'Trends in Alcohol and Illicit Drug-related Diseases', in Office for National Statistics, *The Health of Adult Britain, 1841–1994*, i. London: Stationery Office.

Popay, J. (1992), '"My Health Is All Right, but I'm just Tired All The time"', in H. Roberts (ed.), *Women's Health Matters*, London: Routledge.

Porter, R. (1990), *English Society in the Eighteenth Century*. Harmondsworth: Penguin.

—— (1999). *The Greatest Benefit to Mankind: A Medical History of Humanity from Antiquity to the Present*, London: Fontana.

Prior, L. (1985), 'The Social Construction of Mortality Statistics', *Sociology of Health and Illness*, 7: 165–90.

Resource Allocation Working Party (1976), *Report*. London: HMSO.

Robinson, R., and New, B. (1992), 'Health Economics and Economists in the NHS', *British Medical Journal*, 305: 1361.

Rodberg, L., and Stevenson, G. (1977), 'The Health Care Industry in Advanced Capitalism', *Review of Radical Political Economics*, 9: 104–15.

Rose, D., and O'Reilly, K. (1998), *The ESRC Review of Government Social Classifications*. London: Office for National Statistics.

Rosenberg, W., and Donald, A. (1995), 'Evidence Based Medicine: An Approach to Clinical Problem-solving', *British Medical Journal*, 310: 1122–6.

Rowlingson, K., and Berthoud, R. (1996), *Disability Benefits and Employment: An Evaluation of Disability Working Allowance*, London: Stationery Office.

Royal Commission on the National Health Service (1979), *Report*, London: HMSO.

Sainsbury, D. (1996), *Gender, Equality and Welfare States*, Cambridge: Cambridge University Press.

Salmon, J. W. (1985), 'Profit and Health Care: Trends in Corporatization and Proprietization', *International Journal of Health Services*, 15: 395–418.

Scheff, T. J. (1963), 'Decision Rules, Types of Error, and Their Consequences in Medical Diagnosis', *Behavioural Science*, 8: 97–107.

Secretary of State for Health (1992), *The Health of the Nation*, London: HMSO.

—— (1997), *The New NHS*, London: Stationery Office.

—— (1998a), *Our Healthier Nation*, London: Stationery Office.

Secretary of State for Health (1998b), *A First Class Service: Quality in the New NHS*, London: Stationery Office.

Sedgwick, P. (1982), *PsychoPolitics*, London: Pluto.

Shajahan P. M., and Cavanagh, J. T. (1998), 'Admission for Depression among Men in Scotland, 1980–95: A Retrospective Study', *British Medical Journal*, 316: 1496–7.

Shorter, E. (1997), *A History of Psychiatry*, New York: Wiley.

Shouls, S., Whitehead, M., Burstrom, B., and Diderichson, F. (1999), 'The Health and Socio-economic Circumstances of British Lone Mothers over the Last Two Decades', *Population Trends*, 95, London: ONS.

Silverman, D. (1987), *Communication and Medical Practice: Social Relations in the Clinic*. London: Sage.

Skocpol, T. (1996), *Boomerang: Clinton's Health Security Effort and the Turn of Government in US Politics*. New York: Norton.

Smaje, C. (1995) *Health, 'Race' and Ethnicity: Making Sense of the Evidence*, London: King's Fund.

Spring Rice, M. (1981) [1939], *Working Class Wives: Their Health and Conditions*. London: Virago.

Stacey, M. (1988), *The Sociology of Health and Healing*. London: Unwin Hyman.

Starr, P. (1982), *The Social Transformation of American Medicine*, New York: Basic Books.

Stevenson, T. H. C. (1923), 'The Social Distribution of Mortality from Different Causes in England and Wales 1910–1912', *Biometrika*, 15: 382–400.

Sunday Times Insight Team (1980), *Suffer the Children: The Story of Thalidomide*, London: Futura.

Thoits, P. (1995), 'Stress, Coping and Social Support processes: Where Are We? What Next?', *Journal of Health and Social Behavior*, extra issue, 53–79.

Thomas, C. (1995), 'Domestic Labour and Health: Bringing It All Back Home', *Sociology of Health and Illness*, 17: 328–52.

Tomalin, C. (1997), *Jane Austen*, London: Viking.

Totman, R. (1990), *Mind, Stress and Health*, London: Souvenir Press.

Townsend, P., and Davidson, N. (1988) *The Black Report*, Harmondsworth: Penguin.

——, Phillimore, P., and Beattie, A. (1988), *Health and Deprivation: Inequality and the North*, London: Croom Helm.

Treffers, P., and Pel, M. (1993), 'The rising trend for Caesarian birth', *British Medical Journal*, 307: 1017–18.

Walshe, K., and Ham, C. (1997), 'Who's Acting on the Evidence?', *Health Service Journal*, 107: 22–5.

Warner, R. (1994), *Recovery from Schizophrenia: Psychiatry and Political Economy*, 2nd edn, London: Routledge and Kegan Paul.

Warr, P. (1987), *Work, Unemployment and Mental Health*, Oxford: Clarendon Press.

Webster, C. (1988), *The Health Services since the War*, i: *Problems of Health Care: The National Health Service before 1957*, London: HMSO.

White, A., Nicholaas, G., Foster, K., Browne, F., and Carey, S. (1993), *Health Survey for England 1991*, OPCS Social Survey Division, London: HMSO.

Whitehead, M. (1988), *The Health Divide*, Harmondsworth: Penguin.

—— and Diderichson, F. (1997), 'International Evidence on Social Inequalities in Health', in F. Drever and M. Whitehead (eds.), *Health Inequalities*, London: Stationery Office.

Wilkinson, R. G. (1986a), 'Socio-economic Differences in Mortality: Interpreting the Data on Their Size and Trends', in R. G. Wilkinson (ed.), *Class and Health*, London: Tavistock.

—— (1986b), 'Income and Mortality', in R. G. Wilkinson (ed.), *Class and Health*, London: Tavistock.

—— (1996) *Unhealthy Societies: The Afflictions of Inequality*, London: Routledge

Williams, S. J. (1998), '"Capitalising" on Emotions: Rethinking the Inequalities in Health Debate', *Sociology*, 32: 121–39.

Witz, A. (1992), *Professions and Patriarchy*, London: Routledge.

Wohl, A. (1983), *Endangered Lives: Public Health in Victorian Britain*, London: Dent.

Woodward, J. (1974), *To Do the Sick No Harm: A Study of the British Voluntary Hospital System to 1875*, London: Routledge and Kegan Paul.

World Health Organization (1995), *The World Health Report 1995: Bridging the Gaps*. Geneva: WHO.

Index